Postgraduate Tutorials in General Practice

Edward Warren MB ChB, MRCGP, DRCOG
General Practitioner, Chapelgreen, Sheffield
GP Trainer, Barnsley Vocational Training Scheme

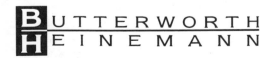
BUTTERWORTH
HEINEMANN

Butterworth-Heinemann
Linacre House, Jordan Hill, Oxford OX2 8DP
A division of Reed Educational and Professional Publishing Ltd

 A member of the Reed Elsevier plc group

OXFORD   BOSTON   JOHANNESBURG
MELBOURNE   NEW DELHI   SINGAPORE

First edition 1995
Reprinted 1997

British Library Cataloguing in Publication Data
Warren, W. E.
    Postgraduate Tutorials in General
    Practice
    I. Title
    362.172

ISBN 0 7506 2164 8

Filmset by Bath Typesetting Ltd, Bath
Printed and bound in Great Britain by Biddles Ltd, Guildford and King's Lynn

Contents

Preface

The literature of general practice is vast and growing. A good excuse is needed by an author who wishes to add to it. The literature not only includes the specialist family care material, but it is arguable that most of the other medical specialties, and biomedicine and sociology in general, are proper study material for the modern general practitioner (GP). Add to this the increasingly important areas of economics and marketing, and the British GP is certainly required to be a new renaissance figure with an intellectual finger in most pies.

With such a vast literature, it is impossible for a trainee to come to terms with it all, and certainly not within the allotted trainee year. Some trainees will react to the task by trying to read everything, starting at page one and carrying on till the end. This approach has all the attractions of painting the Forth Bridge. The job of the trainer is, therefore, to select out the important information as well as to encourage the production of a safe, effective and enthusiastic GP. Indeed, the ability to sort information critically is probably one of the more important skills for a trainee to learn, and one which will make future professional life interesting and tolerable.

I have tried in this book to identify topics which will have relevance to most trainees. This has been helped by my own succession of trainees as it is they who have asked for the topics which appear. The choice of a suitable tutorial topic is informed by the trainee's perceived learning needs, by problems which arise during the day-to-day work, and by the things the trainer thinks the trainee ought to know. Considering the variability of trainees and their work, it is remarkable with what regularity the same topics arise. All the topics in this book have been used at least once in a tutorial setting, and most of them have been used several times.

Each chapter should contain enough material for an hour's discussion. I would suggest that trainer and trainee read it beforehand so at least you are on a level playing field. What happens during the tutorial will then depend on which aspects of the topic seem more interesting or problematic. Some of the most satisfying tutorials I have been involved with have used one or two of the trainee's actual cases and tried to extract relevant teaching points from them. These are often the cases which have stimulated the request for the tutorial in the first place.

Each chapter contains suggested aims for the tutorial, a few relevant statistics, a review of the clinical issues from textbook and recent research, practical management suggestions and discussions of controversial areas. I would not expect anyone to agree completely with the contents of this book, even though I have tried to justify any statistics and controversies with reference to the literature. The aim was to stimulate discussion, not to write a textbook.

The references cited are from articles I happened to have in my filing cabinet, and so there is a heavy emphasis on the most popular and available British literature, and especially on review articles and guidelines published by British authorities. This is deliberate, as it reflects my own reading habits and, I would suggest, those of a majority of 'coal-face' GPs and trainers. If primary sources are required, I recommend consulting the articles cited at the end of each chapter. They are all widely available through medical libraries.

The idea of the traditional tutorial has fallen from favour in educational circles as it does not seem to be a very efficient way of transmitting information. When a mini-lecture occurs, with the trainer bestowing wisdom on the trainee, then the tutorial is probably a complete waste of time. On the other hand, having a specified time in the week when trainer and trainee can have an uninterrupted hour together in discussion can be very effective and satisfying, and is certainly prized by the Joint Committee on Postgraduate Training for General Practice and the trainees themselves. The practical issues of the working day need immediate solutions, and it is not appropriate or fair to the trainee and waiting patients to stop in the middle of a surgery for a 15-minute esoteric discussion. Other times have to be found when the talk can wander in different directions and issues of an ethical or even philosophical nature can be addressed.

I must acknowledge the support I have received in the writing of this book. I would like to thank my publisher Geoff Smaldon, who has been a constant source of encouragement. I am also thankful to the reviewers, Doctors Mike Cohen, Alex Khot and Andrew Polmear. Their comments and criticisms were very necessary and useful, even though they were not always appreciated at the time.

The major acknowledgement must, however, be to my long-suffering wife and children. They have tolerated my obsession with this book for the last year or more without being too critical, and have even allowed me to throw bits of paper all over the floor (which is my idea of a filing system) without more than an occasional muffled cry of anguish. Also I have to include something nice about the family in case I want to do it all over again.

E. W.
Chapelgreen

1

Angina pectoris

Aims

The trainee should:

- Be able to make a clinical diagnosis of angina.
- Know how to structure a management plan for an angina sufferer.
- Be able to counsel the patient deciding between different therapeutic options.

How common is angina?

Angina pectoris is one of the symptomatic manifestations of ischaemic heart disease (IHD). The prevalence of IHD is not known because a large number of sufferers either don't report symptoms or else don't have symptoms. Community studies suggest that the population prevalence of angina is 1.5%, or 2.6% in those aged over 30.[1]

Silent ischaemia

Silent ischaemia is the presence of electrocardiogram (ECG) evidence of ischaemia (usually on exercise) when the patient suffers no symptoms. Its significance is hotly debated, but since it carries a mortality it is suggested that it needs treating like other types of ischaemia.[2]

Another manifestation of IHD is myocardial infarction (MI). In the UK in 1992 there were about 17 000 deaths due to MI.[3] Patients with angina are at risk of having an MI, but there is little correlation between the severity of the angina symptoms and the chance of a subsequent MI.[1]

When populations are screened by ECG, half of all MIs are unrecognized, and a quarter cause no symptoms.[2]

Why does angina happen?

Angina occurs when insufficient blood gets through to the myocardium. There are two possible reasons for this:

- Inadequate blood flow or blood quality.
- Excessive myocardial demand.

The usual reason for inadequate flow is the narrowing of the coronary arteries by atheroma or other reasons, though a similar effect is produced by poor cardiac output, for example because of aortic stenosis.

In patients with anaemia, the blood may not be able to carry sufficient oxygen for the needs of the myocardium.

The blood supply will be able to sustain myocardial work up to a threshold, but beyond this, symptoms of angina will occur. This leads to the universal finding in stable angina that symptoms are brought on by exertion and relieved by rest, and indeed this is the way in which stable and unstable angina can be distinguished.

Excessive myocardial requirement for blood can be produced by hypertension, exercise or valvular heart disease. It is quite uncommon for this of itself to produce angina, and there is usually coexisting arterial narrowing which only begins to produce symptoms when myocardial demand increases.

How can you diagnose angina?

The diagnosis of angina is made mainly from the history.

Pain

Typically the sufferer will have episodes of central chest pain of a tight or crushing nature. The patient will often use a clenched fist when describing the character of the pain.[4] There may be radiation to the inside of the left arm, or sometimes both arms, or to the neck or jaw. Sometimes pain may be experienced in the radiation sites but not in the chest.

Breathlessness

This may occur with the pain, or alone.

Exertion

The symptoms of angina come on with exertion of a physical or sometimes emotional nature, and are relieved by rest. Lesser degrees of exercise may just bring on breathlessness and not the pain. Occasionally it may be possible to 'walk through' the pain, but usually it is only rest which helps the symptoms abate.

Other provocations

Cold weather, wind, and just having eaten a heavy meal all lower the angina threshold. People with angina often alter their habits to minimize the number of attacks. This may create the impression that the angina is 'cured'.

Questions to ask:[4]

- Where is the pain?
- Where does it go?
- What brings it on?
- What relieves it?
- What does it feel like?

What are the types of angina?

Stable angina

Stable angina occurs when symptoms gradually increase with time. There is a gradual build-up of plaque in the coronary arteries with consequent gradual reduction in lumen diameter. Symptoms always begin at roughly the same level of exertion. Cold weather or a meal or coexistent emotional strain may lower this threshold.

Unstable angina

Unstable angina is where the intensity of the angina and the provocation needed to induce it vary considerably. Thrombus has probably formed, and this produces various vasoactive substances which contract the artery. The dynamic relationship between the build-up of thrombus and the contraction of the coronary arteries gives rise to the fluctuating symptoms.

Crescendo angina

Crescendo angina occurs when angina becomes progressively worse so that there is pain at rest or on minimal exertion.

Angina with normal coronary arteries

This rare type of angina produces typical symptoms, but they can arise at any time and are not related to exercise. The reason is thought to be excessive spasm of the muscles round the coronary arteries. Unlike other types of angina, women are more likely to be affected than men (5:1) and, though the prognosis is excellent, more than 70% of women have persisting symptoms and 50% are disabled by them.[5]

Is treatment needed urgently?

Stable angina

Stable angina is a risk factor for MI, but does not mean that such an event is imminent. Treatment is dictated by the need to reduce symptoms and improve exercise tolerance. There is little to be gained by obtaining an urgent cardiology opinion, and such a strategy would almost certainly generate anxiety.

Unstable angina

In unstable angina the severity of the symptoms and the provocation needed to produce them vary considerably. There may be a history of stable angina, and some patients pass back from unstable to stable angina. If unstable angina is diagnosed, then there is a real chance of an imminent MI. The patient needs an early assessment, usually as a result of an urgent outpatient visit.

Crescendo angina

Crescendo angina is diagnosed if the angina is progressive so that the pains have worsened in severity, maybe coming on at rest, and are unrelieved by nitrates, or the frequency of nitrate use has rapidly increased. The sudden worsening of symptoms may lead to a clinical diagnosis of MI, and the absence of a rise in enzyme levels may be the only indication that an MI has not occurred.

After an episode of crescendo angina, 8–13% of patients will have an acute MI within 1 month, and 8–15% will be dead inside a year.[6] Urgent admission is needed.

In 80% of cases the problem can be managed medically. Antithrombotic medication in the form of aspirin 150–300 mg/day reduces the chance of MI and death by 50%.

The initial work-up of a new case of angina

Examination

The examination of the patient with angina is usually normal.[4]

The chance of a patient benefiting from treatment of their IHD risk factors depends on the overall risk: high-risk patients have most to gain. The patient with angina has existing vascular pathology, and so it is reasonable to look for other treatable risk factors.

Cigarette smoking
Look for nicotine-stained fingers and smell for smoke. Ask about smoking habits.

Hyperlipidaemia
A premature arcus senilis (under 40 years) or xanthomata or xanthelasmata on the hands, knees, eyelids or elbows suggests abnormal lipid levels.

Peripheral vascular disease
Femoral and carotid arteries may yield bruits.

Blood pressure
Hypertension is a risk factor for IHD, and the risk can be reduced with treatment. Hypertension also increases the heart's workload, and so lowers the angina threshold.

Examination of the heart and lungs should be done, looking for evidence of a valve lesion, left heart failure or anaemia.

Investigation

Investigations are sometimes but not always helpful.

- A resting ECG is normal in over half of patients with angina,[4] and obtaining a normal ECG in a patient with chest pain has very unreliable prognostic power.
- An exercise ECG is more helpful but many GPs do not have open access to this service. An exercise test is only 85% sensitive in detecting patients likely to gain from surgery.[4] However, the test is 85% specific, and so it is a very good way of excluding non-anginal chest pain.
- Problems in the form of ventricular fibrillation occur in about 1 in 5000 tests.[4] Digoxin should be stopped 7 days before a test,

and β-blockers 48 hours before, as these drugs may give rise to false-positive and false-negative results respectively.
- Haemoglobin estimation is useful to rule out those with anaemia.
- Serum cholesterol should be assayed in the under 55s.[7]

Is the diagnosis in doubt?

Nitrate trial

When the diagnosis is uncertain and the patient is not too severely affected, then a trial of nitrate can help clarify the picture.[7] Sublingual glyceryl trinitrate in a dose of 500 μg can be prescribed, or bought if the patient is not exempt from prescription charges as the cost will be less. The tablets should be used when symptoms occur, and if relief is obtained within 2–3 minutes it may be concluded that the pain is caused by angina.[8]

At follow-up 7–10 days later the effect of treatment can be assessed, and the diagnosis confirmed. Longer-term management is dictated by the success of symptom control and the limitation of function.

This is an appropriate course of action where:

- Symptoms are mild.
- Referral is not being considered.
- Other considerations make surgery unlikely.

Remember, however, that glyceryl trinitrate also helps oesophageal pain.

Exercise ECG

In some centres exercise ECG tests are available to GPs on an open access basis, but this facility is not universal. As well as confirming the diagnosis, the exercise ECG also gives a good indication of which patients might benefit from surgery.

What can you tell the patient with angina?

A number of different pathological processes may contribute to the angina, and this explains the different types of angina which occur.[7] In all cases there is damage to the intima of coronary arteries and the deposition of cholesterol plaques.

As cholesterol is deposited in the walls of the artery, an atheromatous plaque builds up which narrows the lumen. Once the lumen gets to a critical size, there is a chance that thrombus may form.

The intima over the surface of plaques has a 'crazy paving' configuration rather than the linear arrangement found in normal intima. This tends to disrupt blood flow and cause turbulence, increasing the chance of thrombus formation.

Just below the tip of a plaque is a junction between the atheroma and the fibrous tip. Shear stresses from blood flow may break into the epithelium at this weaker point, causing turbulence and hence thrombus formation.

What are the treatment options?

In all cases

Smoking
Risk factors for angina are the same as those for MI. Smoking should be counselled against. For cigarette smokers this is by far the most important part of the treatment.

Dietary advice
This will be appropriate for the obese. Patients under 55 should have their cholesterol levels checked[7] and advised accordingly.

Exercise
Exercise is to be encouraged – regular gentle exercise, preferably falling short of inducing symptoms. Twenty minutes of exercise three times a week in the form of swimming, moderate walking (3 miles an hour) or similar will bring about an improvement in general fitness and exercise tolerance. Patients with unstable angina need rest, but this group will have been referred anyway and treatment organized by the specialist. If the unstable angina has reverted to stable angina, then exercise can be advised.

Raised blood pressure
Raised blood pressure should be treated. The presence of angina indicates existing vascular pathology and so treatment even in the mildly hypertensive is likely to be beneficial.

Anxieties
Anxieties should be addressed. A diagnosis of angina can make an

enormous psychological impact. Some people react by becoming 'professional' sufferers. Life becomes dominated by the angina, self-help groups are joined, diet and exercise regimes are obsessively followed. There is a tendency to have excessive contacts with the medical services, often for trivial reasons, in order to confirm the continuing success of their fight against the disease. A constant testing of exercise tolerance may occur. The potential for disappointment in this group is considerable, but at least they follow medical advice closely.

Other patients may be devastated by the diagnosis, and convinced of their complete disability and imminent demise. In this group there is also a complete change in lifestyle, but this time towards inactivity and despair. Frank depression may occur.

Most patients eventually get over their initial shock and adjust to pursue a sensible change in their habits and activities. A compromise is struck between improved habits, the use of medication and some limitations of activity. This is probably the most healthy response and is to be encouraged.

Medication: what are the choices?

Most patients with angina pectoris are treated with β-blockers or calcium channel blockers. Short-acting nitrates retain an important role both when chest pain has occurred and for prophylactic use before exertion. Nitrates are sometimes used as sole therapy, especially in elderly patients with infrequent symptoms.

When one type of drug has been used in full dose and the symptoms are not controlled, another should be added. If symptoms then come under control it is sometimes possible gradually to withdraw the first agent to see if it is still having an effect. Most angina sufferers also carry a nitrate on a 'just in case' basis as well. If two types of drug in full dosage fail to control the angina then a third agent may be added, but the evidence for the third agent giving extra benefits is lacking.[5] At this point a referral should be considered.

Aspirin

The use of small doses of aspirin has been shown to reduce the rate of MI in both stable (a 34% reduction) and unstable angina.[1] A dose of 150 mg/day is recommended, though a dose of 75 mg has been used in many of the trials with good effect. The smaller dose is recommended in those patients who are intolerant of the larger dose. There is also now available an enteric-coated 75 mg preparation.

Nitrates

Nitrates have been used medically for 100 years and are the mainstay of drug treatment. When used systemically they cause arterial and venous dilatation, thus reducing preload and afterload. There is also a minor direct effect on coronary arteries, especially where spasm is a problem.[9] This leads to a decrease in cardiac workload, and a slightly improved perfusion of the myocardium.

Given sublingually, nitrates cause an initial arterial dilatation, and a subsequent venodilation. Used orally, transdermally or intravenously the predominant action is venodilation.[10]

Side-effects of nitrates include flushing, headaches and postural hypotension. These are entirely consistent with the mode of action of the drug and indicate that it is having an effect.

For acute use, sublingual glyceryl trinitrate has a peak action in 4–8 minutes and is effective for 10–30 minutes.[10] It is very cheap, but the tablet is unstable and only lasts 8 weeks once the bottle is open. Any side-effects can be minimized by spitting out the tablet as soon as symptomatic relief is obtained. The initial dose is 500–1000 µg (1–2 tablets), but the smaller 300 µg tablets can be used if side-effects are a persisting problem.

Sublingual isosorbide dinitrate is an alternative, but it is more expensive and takes 15–60 minutes to start working. However, its duration of action is longer, at 45–120 minutes,[10] and the tablet is more stable, making it useful in the patient who needs only occasional treatment. A dose of 5–10 mg is used.

For long-term use, the choice of oral therapies is between isosorbide in its dinitrate (ISDM) or mononitrate (ISMN) forms. ISDM is cheaper, and is metabolized to the mononitrate. However, it only works for 2–6 hours, so has to be given four times a day.[11] It is also metabolized in the liver so that blood levels are unpredictable. The dose is from 30 mg up to a maximum of 120 mg day.

ISMN is now more widely used. Its longer duration of action (6–10 hours) means that it can be used twice a day. Once-daily formulations are more expensive. The starting dose in those who have not had nitrates before is 10 mg twice a day, or 40 mg twice a day in the previously exposed.[11] This can be increased to 60 mg twice a day if required.

Transdermal glyceryl trinitrate can also last up to 24 hours and avoids the first-pass effect. The metabolism of nitrates in the liver can lead to unreliable blood levels. By direct absorption through the skin, transdermal preparations avoid this and so theoretically the angina control should be better. This is not borne out clinically in most cases. Products are expensive, and sometimes topical sensitivity develops to the drug or plaster. Strengths of 5 and 10 mg are available.

Sublingual glyceryl trinitrate sprays are no more effective dose-for-dose than the tablets,[12] but the shelf-life of the spray is much longer. They are more expensive than the glyceryl trinitrate tablets.

Tolerance to nitrates is a problem with chronic use of any formulation. It may happen within 24 hours of starting treatment.[10] A drug-free period of 8 hours a day is recommended, or the drug will be less effective. The once-daily formulations are designed to 'run out', so that for several hours the body can wash out the nitrate. Users of the patches are recommended to take them off at bedtime. In angina with normal coronary arteries, the symptoms are often worse at night, in which case the washout period is better in the day.

β-Blockers

These drugs work by reducing the contractility and rate of the heart, thus reducing work. In addition they reduce exercise-induced vasoconstriction, and so are particularly useful in effort-related angina.[13]

There is no good evidence that one agent is generally any better than the rest in treating angina, though some patients respond better to one drug than another. Cardioselective agents such as atenolol are preferred on theoretical grounds.

Gastrointestinal disturbance, fatigue, cold extremities, erectile impotence and sleep disturbance because of vivid (but not necessarily unpleasant) dreams are common side-effects.

β-Blockers should not be used in asthmatics unless there is no alternative. Heart failure also contraindicates their use, and the concurrent use of verapamil is particularly likely to precipitate heart failure in the patient with IHD.

The clinical effect is related to dosage. A reasonable starting dose of propranolol is 40 mg twice a day, but this can rise to 240 mg a day in divided doses if necessary. The equivalent dose for atenolol is 50–100 mg day.[11]

Calcium channel blockers

By blocking calcium influx into smooth muscle, these agents have an effect on blood vessel walls, and a direct effect on the myocardium. As well as reducing afterload, they also improve myocardial perfusion and reduce myocardial contractility.[13]

There is considerable variation in the different agents in the extent to which they produce cardiac and vascular effects. All may precipitate heart failure, and all may produce flushing, headaches, gastrointestinal disturbance, bradycardia, hypotension and ankle oedema.

Nifedipine and the other dihydropyridines work mainly on peripheral blood vessels and can be given in a dose of 10–20 mg (5 mg in the elderly) three times a day. Amlodipine is twice as expensive but only needs to be given once a day in a dose of 5–10 mg.

Verapamil and diltiazem also reduce heart rate, and should not be used with β-blockers. Verapamil has a significant negatively inotropic effect and so is particularly likely to cause hypotension and heart failure. The dose for verapamil is 80–120 mg three times a day, and for diltiazem 60–120 mg three times a day (or start with 60 mg twice a day in the elderly).

What are the aims of treatment?

Exercise is good for hearts, whether they have angina or not. Good control in angina means that the sufferer should be able to do the things he or she wants to do. The medication is not analgesic, and no harm comes from long-term use. Exertion, whether recreational or due to work, may induce symptoms, but this should suggest a change in therapy rather than a need to give up the exertion. When all has been done, however, some patients will need to give up working because of their angina.

Angina of itself is not a reason to stop driving, and does not need reporting to the licensing authority unless the angina is brought on by driving.[14]

A further aim of treatment is the prevention of other vascular events such as stroke and MI. Any IHD risk factors identified during the course of investigating and treating the angina should be addressed with vigour. In general, benefit from treating these other risks is greater than if the patient had not already had evidence of vascular pathology.

Which patients will benefit from referral?

In the following instances, referral is required:

- There is doubt about the diagnosis and further advice is needed.
- Failure of two-drug treatment. The patient may need further investigation to confirm the diagnosis, or may be a candidate for

surgery.
- Crescendo angina is diagnosed or suspected. Admission or urgent outpatient appointment is needed.
- Patients who may benefit in terms of function or mortality from surgery. The young or functionally young are more likely candidates.

What can you tell your patient about surgery for angina?

Surgery should not be considered until optimal conservative treatment has proved unsuccessful.

Coronary angiography is a necessary precursor to all types of surgery. It is a relatively minor test in surgical terms, but there is a small but definite mortality (0.13%) connected with it. The femoral artery is usually approached via the right groin and the resulting wound is in just the right place to be sore and get infected. There is also a risk of femoral haematoma (0.25%).[15]

Surgery will nearly always help the symptoms of angina. However, whether it will make the chance of an MI or death less likely is not certain. Some groups of patients clearly benefit in terms of mortality, but others do no better than they would on medical treatment.

Coronary artery bypass grafting (CABG)

This operation involves a thoracotomy and about 10–12-day stay in hospital. It can be used in a wide range of circumstances, but in one- or two-vessel disease it is no better than drug therapy in terms of long-term survival.

The operative mortality is 2%.[15] The major longer-term problem is restenosis of the graft. If the internal mammary artery is used for the graft, then 95% will be patent at 10 years. This compares with 50% if a leg vein is used.[15] After surgery, 90% of patients are free of angina at 1 year.[15]

Percutaneous transluminal coronary angioplasty

This is done by passing a balloon into a stenosed coronary artery, then inflating it so that the plaque is squashed. It is a much less invasive procedure than CABG and hospital stay is at most 2 days. In 80–90% of cases there is improvement in symptoms and exercise capacity.[16]

Percutaneous transluminal coronary angioplasty is best used where the stenosis is short, but the procedure can be repeated at a number of sites at the same operation. Restenosis occurs in 17–40% of cases, usually after 3–4 months. Mortality from the procedure is about 1%. In 2% a coronary thrombosis is caused by the procedure, and a further 2% need urgent CABG.[16]

What are the other causes of chest pain?

Any structure in the chest can give rise to pain, and there may also be referred pain from the spine.

- There may be a history of reflux and dyspepsia, which points to an oesophageal cause for the pain. Of the organic causes of chest pain, however, reflux is the hardest one to distinguish from angina on clinical grounds.
- Pleuritic pain is different in character to angina, and will be brought on by breathing and movement rather than exertion. There may be other respiratory symptoms.
- Chest wall pain is stabbing and intermittent and may be provoked by movement or particular activities. There may well be sites on the chest wall which are tender to palpation. Costochondritis causes one or a number of tender spots over the costochondral cartilages.
- Functional chest pain is not uncommon, and is difficult to treat because of the anxiety it generates. Such may be the worry that the patient hyperventilates, which of itself gives rise to breathlessness, increased anxiety and crushing central chest pain. These new symptoms serve to reinforce the 'serious' nature of the disease.

The typical patient presenting with non-cardiac but worrying chest pain is the young fit male with no tradition of ill health or bodily discomfort. Risk factors for ischaemia are absent, and indeed those patients who present are probably more likely not to smoke, eat or drink to excess, and are more likely to undertake healthy behaviour such as regular exercise. A worried spouse is often in attendance or has instigated the consultation.

Sometimes it is possible to implicate muscle tension when explaining the pain. It is helpful if the patient's fears can be relieved without recourse to further investigation, as this raises the suggestion that the pain may be serious, and the delay in getting the results back further increases anxiety. Though not investigating is objectively desirable, in most cases it will be necessary to run a few tests to reinforce your advice and counselling.

References

1. Angina pectoris – a review of treatment. *MeRec Bull* 1994; **5**: 29–32
2. Campbell S. Silent myocardial ischaemia. *Br Med J* 1988; **297**: 751–2
3. *Coronary Heart Disease Statistics*. London: British Heart Foundation. 1994
4. Jackson G. Stable angina. *The Practitioner* 1993; **237**: 922–4
5. Jackson G. New treatments for angina. *Update* 1994; **49**: 245–50
6. *Unstable angina. Factfile*. London: British Heart Foundation. 1993
7. Gershlick AH. Investigation and management of angina. *Update* 1992; **45**: 19–28
8. *Is it Angina? Factfile*. London: British Heart Foundation. 1991
9. Nitrates for angina pectoris (part 1). *MeReC Bull* 1992; **3**: 37–40
10. *Nitrates in Angina. Factfile*. London: British Heart Foundation. 1989
11. *British National Formulary* 27. London: London: British Medical Association/ Royal Pharmaceutical Society of Great Britain
12. Glyceryl trinitrate for angina: tablets or spray? *Drug Ther Bull* 1992; **30**: 93–94
13. Purcell H & Mulcahy D. What action should I take after diagnosing angina? *Monitor Weekly* 1993; **6**: 21–3
14. *Driving and the Heart. Factfile*. London: British Heart Foundation 1992
15. Shapiro LM. Angina pectoris: patient assessment. *Update* 1993; **47**: 798–805
16. Angioplasty in the management of coronary artery disease. *Drug Ther Bull* 1993; **31**: 45–47

For a concise *aide-mémoire* see Khot & Polmear *Practical General Practice*, 2nd edn. Oxford: Butterworth-Heinemann, 1992, pp 104–6.

2

Melanoma and the general practitioner

Aims

The trainee should:

- Be able to recall the clinical features of a melanoma, and know which pigmented lesions need to be to referred.
- Know the natural history of the mole.
- Be able to advise patients on preventive strategies for melanoma.

Why is melanoma important?

The UK Cancer Registry during 1990 received reports on 3119 new cases of melanoma and 1200 deaths from the disease. Each GP with an average list size can therefore expect to see 1 new case of melanoma every 10 years, and the overall population incidence of new cases is 1 in 20 000 per year.[1]

There are roughly 6–7 cases of melanoma in women for every 4 in men.[2] Melanoma accounts for 1.2% of all cancers, and it is the 15th commonest cancer in women and the 17th commonest in men.[1]

Some patients inherit a predisposition to develop melanoma. In the dysplastic naevus syndrome (see later), each individual carries a sevenfold increased risk of the disease, but if there is also a family history of melanoma, this risk rises to 500-fold.[1]

The incidence of melanoma has increased over recent years in all white-skinned populations. The best UK statistics are available for Scotland where there is a particular problem with melanoma, thought to be due to genetic factors. The Scottish Melanoma Group have been gathering data since 1979. From 1979 to 1989 there was an 80% rise in the incidence of new cases.[3] The increase in incidence is matched almost exactly by the increase in package holidays to sunnier countries.

The median age for a diagnosis of malignant melanoma is 53 years.[1] Occurrence in young people is very rare but not unknown.

The overall chance of a patient in England and Wales who is diagnosed as having a melanoma being alive 5 years later is 75% for women and 52% for men.[2] Survival rates are much better for the lesions which are thinner at diagnosis, and though it would seem logical that thin lesions are the earlier stages of thicker lesions, there is no conclusive evidence that early detection of melanoma confers any reduction in mortality.[2]

Once a patient develops disseminated melanoma, the 5-year chance of survival is under 5%, and the median survival time is only 6 months.[1]

What happens to a normal mole?

Naevus is the Latin for birth mark. The components of a naevus, though normal, are abnormally mixed. An excess of blood vessels produces a strawberry naevus or port wine stain. Those with an excess of pigment cells (melanocytes) are called moles.

Melanocytes are found in the basal cell layer of the epidermis, and contain the pigment melanin. Moles are clusters of melanocytes, and are commoner in fair-skinned peoples. Their number is prenatally determined, though there may be other factors involved so that, for instance, they are commoner in children who have had chemotherapy.[4]

The mole's progress

Most moles are not present at birth but appear in the second and third decades. There are usually 20–30 on a fair-skinned person.

1. At first they are dark, flat and up to 1 cm across, and the melanocytes cluster round the dermoepidermal junction – the so-called junctional naevus.
2. They then grow and spread into the dermis to form a compound naevus, which becomes slightly raised.
3. Later the mole stops growing and the melanocytes sink into the dermis, leaving a papule.
4. In later life the mole may disappear, leaving a fibrous nodule.
5. In adolescence, a mole may develop a white halo and disappear quite quickly – the halo naevus.

Other types of mole

1. The true *congenital mole*, which is often very big (e.g. the bathing trunk naevus), dark, hairy, and present at or just after birth is particularly prone to malignant change. The risk of malignant change is around 3% in such a mole.[5] Removal of the lesion (where this is practical) at around 10 years is often recommended.

2. Unusual or *dysplastic moles* (for example, with irregular edges or colouring or size over 3 mm) are also more likely to undergo malignant change. In the familial condition of dysplastic naevus syndrome, an autosomal dominant condition with incomplete penetrance, malignant change is common and often multiple. The individual will usually be freckled and fair-skinned. There will be three or more naevi of a dysplastic nature, as well as at least 30 others. There is often a family history of melanoma.

Which patients are at risk from melanoma?

Up to 10% of melanomas are thought to be associated with inherited characterisics.[2] As well as those patients who have already had a melanoma or who have a family history of melanoma, other groups are at increased risk.[1] Most of the risk factors for melanoma are unavoidable (the exception is sun exposure):

• Patients with fair skin, blue eyes, freckles and a tendency to sunburn.
• A history of severe sunburn in childhood.
• Celtic (Scottish or Irish) ancestry, especially in patients who have moved to live in Australia, New Zealand or southern USA.
• Dysplastic naevus syndrome.
• Patients with a congenital naevus.

How can you spot a melanoma?

Suspicious lesions need to be biopsied and dealt with as early as possible. Delays of 6 months or more between the patient noticing a possible problem and the eventual biopsy are not uncommon. Some of this delay is because the patients do not present themselves. Further delay is, however, caused by poor referral practices: in one study[6] 22% of referral letters did not mention pigmentation and 56% did not request an urgent outpatient appointment.

Of the suspicious lesions seen by British dermatologists, around 5% turn out to have undergone malignant change. In the USA and the Netherlands, where patients have open access to skin clinics, the corresponding figures are 0.4 and 0.2%.[3]

Over 90% of melanomas can be recognized by experienced observers, though this falls to 50% in the inexperienced.[1] The definitive diagnosis is only made after biopsy.

With minor surgery payments, more and more melanomas are being removed by GPs without suspicions being raised as to the histology. This emphasizes the need to submit all excised skin lesions for analysis, especially pigmented ones.

What are the important clinical features?

Various checklists have been produced to identify malignant melanomas. This one[3] was derived from work done in Glasgow by the Scottish Melanoma Group. Common clinical features are divided into major and minor.

Major features

- Change in size.
- Change in colour.
- Change in shape.

Minor features are only relevant in combination with at least one major feature:

- Inflammation.
- Crusting or bleeding.
- Sensory change, i.e. itching.
- Size over 7 mm in diameter.

Urgent referral is needed if one or more of the major features is present. Further delays in treatment result if the urgency of the referral is not indicated to the dermatologist.

A review published in 1994[7] showed that if the diagnosis of melanoma is made on the basis of just one of the features, then the sensitivity is 100% and the specificity is 37%. If two major features are needed for the diagnosis, then sensitivity is 65% and specificity is 96%. A diagnostic test for GPs needs a high sensitivity. A low specificity is more of a problem for the dermatologist.

What are the different types of melanoma?

Superficial spreading melanoma

These constitute 50% of the total and are the commonest type. Women are affected twice as often as men. In women they usually occur on the legs, and in men on the trunk and particularly the back. There is a spreading macular lesion. They usually occur after age 40 and commonly between 40 and 60.

Nodular melanoma

These form 25% of the total. This is a much faster-growing lesion which develops nodules and ulcers at an early stage. They may be red, grey or black in colour, and 5% are colourless – the amelanotic melanoma. The prognosis is poor.

Lentigo maligna melanoma

These form 15% of the total. This is a slow-growing brown macule, usually on the face, which may have been present for years. It becomes nodular as it changes to a malignant phase. An older age group is affected, usually over 60.

Acral melanoma

This makes up 6% of the total. It occurs on the extremities (finger ends, under nails, soles of feet). It often presents late. It affects an older age group.

What can you say to a patient with a melanoma?

Once the diagnosis is confirmed, the patient may turn to you for advice and support. It is important to have an idea of what the patient can expect from treatment. Counselling can only be effective if supported by trust, honesty and accurate information.

The primary treatment of melanoma is by wide excision, with a 1 cm margin for thin lesions and a 3 cm margin for thicker ones. It may therefore be necessary to graft the skin deficit left by surgery. Neither chemotherapy nor radiotherapy at this stage helps the prognosis, and so the patient will be followed-up only by regular clinical examination for at least 5 and usually 10 years before a cure is assumed. First recurrence after 5 years is uncommon.[8]

Overall the prognosis is dependent on the thickness of the melanoma at biopsy. This is the Breslow thickness.[8]

5-year survival:

- Under 1.5 mm = 91%
- 1.5–3.5 mm = 67%
- Over 3.5 mm = 38%

Local recurrences are treated by further excisions. Metastatic and node-positive lesions may benefit from further surgery, and there is also evidence of benefit from chemotherapy. Palliative radiotherapy can also be useful.

Can melanoma be prevented?

Deaths from melanoma can either be avoided by primary prevention, or by the early recognition and treatment of lesions.

An initiative in Scotland began in 1985 to secure early recognition of melanomas by patients and GPs. This led to an increase of 278% in the referral of suspicious lesions to dermatology clinics and a 131% increase in the number of melanomas confirmed. The number of melanomas of thickness under 1.5 mm rose from 38 to 54%. From 1988 onwards the mortality from melanoma began to fall, but only in women.[9] This improvement has occurred, however, in the context of a high-risk population, specific educational initiatives for doctors and patients, and special pigmented lesion clinics being set up. Its success if applied to the rest of the UK cannot be assumed.[2]

Exposure to ultraviolet radiation is the only known risk factor for melanoma which is alterable.

The *Health of the Nation* has highlighted skin cancer as a key area for prevention. Melanoma constitutes 11% of all skin cancers. The target is to halt the year-on-year increase in the numbers of skin cancers by 2005.[10] The suggested means of doing this are:

- To increase the number of people who are aware of their own skin cancer risk factors and in the light of that knowledge:
- To persuade people at high risk to avoid excessive exposure to the sun and artificial sources of ultraviolet radiation, for themselves and for their children, through the adoption of appropriate avoidance behaviour and sun protection measures.
- To secure an alteration in people's attitude to a tanned appearance.

How damaging is sun exposure?

Unlike other forms of skin cancer where total cumulative exposure to sunlight is a risk factor, the risk of getting melanoma is related more closely to episodes of sunburn.[1] People who work outdoors are less likely to get a melanoma than the indoor worker who spends leisure time in the sun.

In a 1994 review of the literature,[11] it was concluded that adults who recall numerous episodes of sunburn are two to three times more likely to get a melanoma. This effect is independent of the skin type of the sufferer. In addition, episodes of sunburn in children under the age of 15 confer a fivefold increased risk of melanoma in later life. Around 40% of children in the UK have an episode of sunburn at least once a year, and this nearly always occurs in the UK.[12] Melanoma is rare (but not unknown) in children, so the effect may be to produce susceptibility in the patient for later years.

Estimating the risk of melanoma has to take into account the fact that melanoma is a rare disease. Quoting a fivefold increase in risk makes it sound as though any exposure to sunlight will lead to a melanoma. However, the fivefold change in risk is from about 1 in 20 000 to 1 in 4000, or 0.005% to 0.025% which still constitutes a very small risk.

Will a public awareness programme work?

An initiative in Australia called SunSmart aimed over 3 years to alter the public's attitudes towards sun exposure. An increase in perceived vulnerability to skin cancer was achieved, and there was an increase from 39 to 51% in the numbers of people who did not desire any degree of suntan.[2]

As episodes of sunburn in childhood seem to be an important risk for melanoma, it may well be 20 or 30 years before the effects of reducing sun exposure are translated into fewer melanomas. At least as far as melanoma is concerned, the *Health of the Nation* target is unlikely to be achieved.[13]

What can you tell the worried holidaymaker?

Since Coco Chanel emerged from her cruise with a 'healthy tan' in 1930, GPs and dermatologists have been fighting a losing battle with the package-tour industry.

The Royal College of Dermatologists has suggested a four-point programme for reducing sun exposure:[14] avoid the noonday sun; seek natural shade; wear clothing and hats; and use a broad-spectrum sunscreen with a sun protection factor (SPF) of 15 or above.

Suncreams only last for 2 hours and have to be regularly reapplied, especially to areas often forgotten, like the back of the neck. They also wash off. SPF 10 means that you can stay in the sun 10 times longer than if you had no protection. SPF only indicates protection from ultraviolet B (UVB) light – this is important as UVB is 1000 times more likely to cause burns than UVA, but there is more UVA in sunlight. There is no internationally agreed standard to denote protection from UVA.

High SPF creams can be prescribed under Advisory Committee on Borderline Substances regulations, but only in photosensitive patients with a skin condition from a specific qualifying list. Sunburn in a normal skin is not one of these qualifying conditions.

SPF 10 is all right for easily tanning skin, but in the fair-skinned an SPF of 15 or over is required.[15]

Clothes are a much better protection against sunlight than creams. Loose and light clothing works best, not forgetting collars and sleeves.

Due to ozone depletion, the amount of ultraviolet light in sunlight is increasing. UVC, which is even more damaging than UVB, is usually completely absorbed by the ozone layer. The maximum levels of ultraviolet light in UK sunlight are found in May and June. Even the sun levels found in the UK can cause problems.

In hotter climates, it is best to avoid the sun for the hours either side of midday, from 11 a.m. to 3 p.m. The shadow rule can help: if your shadow is bigger than you, then the sun is safer.

References

1. Taylor A and Gore M. Melanoma: detection and management. *Update* 1994; **48**: 209–19
2. Austoker J. Melanoma: prevention and early diagnosis. *Br Med J* 1994; **308**: 1682–6
3. MacKie RM. Clinical recognition of early invasive malignant melanoma. *Br Med J* 1990; **301**: 1005–6
4. Jamieson JA. Moles. *Maternal Child Health* 1992; 294–98
5. Newton JA. Sun and skin: the epidemiology of melanoma. *Maternal Child Health* 1993; **18**: 378–81
6. Dunkley MP and Morris AM. Cutaneous malignant melanoma: an audit of the diagnostic process. *Ann R Coll Surg Engl* 1991; **73**: 248–52
7. Healsmith MF, Bourke JF, Osborne JF *et al*. An evaluation of the revised seven

point check list for the early diagnosis of cutaneous malignant melanoma. *Br J Dermatol* 1994; **130**: 48–50

8. Malignant melanoma of the skin. *Drug Ther Bull* 1988; **26**: 73–75
9. MacKie RM and Hole D. Audit of public education campaign to encourage earlier detection of malignant melanoma. *Br Med J* 1992; **304**: 1012–15
10. Secretary of State for Health. *Health of the Nation: A Strategy for Health in England.* London: HMSO. 1992
11. Marks R and Whiteman D. Sunburn and melanoma: how strong is the evidence? *Br Med J* 1994; **308**: 75–6
12. Jarrett P, Sharp C and McLelland J. Protection of children by their mother against sunburn. *Br Med J* 1993; **306**: 1448
13. Marks R. Primary prevention of skin cancer. *Br Med J* 1994; **309**: 28–56
14. United Kingdom Skin Cancer Prevention Working Party. *Consensus Statement.* London: British Association of Dermatologists. 1994
15. Ratnavel RC and Norris PG. Sunscreens and their medical uses. *Prescribers' J* 1993; **33**: 63–70

3

The management of stroke and its consequences

Aims

The trainee should:

- Be able to make an urgent assessment of a stroke victim and plan acute care appropriately.
- Be able to assess and plan care for the chronic needs of the patient and carers.
- Have knowledge of the preventive strategies available.

Definitions

Stroke

According to the World Health Organization, a cerebrovascular accident (CVA) or stroke is:

> Rapidly developing clinical signs of focal loss of cerebral function, with symptoms lasting more than 24 hours or leading to death, with no apparent cause other than of vascular origin.[1]

Transient ischaemic attack

A transient ischaemic attack (TIA) is defined as:

> An acute loss of focal cerebral function with symptoms lasting less than 24 hours with no apparent cause other than that of vascular origin.[2]

Facts and figures

About 100 000 people each year in the UK suffer a first stroke. Of these, 25 000 are under 65 years old, 29 000 are between 65 and 74, and the rest are over 75.[3] Stroke is a disease of old age, and with numbers of the very elderly expected to rise in the future, the incidence of stroke will surely also rise.

More strokes occur in patients who have had a previous episode, so the overall incidence of stroke is 2 per 1000 per year.

Putting this into primary care terms, each GP will on average have four new strokes a year to deal with, as well as 12–15 patients with a past history of stroke.[4]

In addition, 25 000 people a year suffer a TIA.[5]

A total of 64 000 deaths each year are due to stroke, representing 12% of all deaths. Stroke is the third commonest cause of death. In the under-65s, there are 5000 deaths (or 5% of all deaths), and in the 65–74s 11 000 (or 9% of all). Both the incidence and the chance of dying of a stroke rise with age.[3]

Over the past 20 years there has been a reduction in mortality from stroke of between 2 and 7% each year.[3] The beginning of this reduction predates the widespread interest in treating hypertension.

Twenty-four per cent of the severely disabled in a community will be stroke victims.[6] Stroke care consumes around 5% of all NHS resources.[1]

What to do when called to a possible stroke

It is important to attend promptly. The patient and carers will be distressed at such a sudden occurrence of severe symptoms. In a minority of cases it may also be medically useful to see the patient as soon as possible. Strokes, like other thrombotic events, are commoner in the hours just after waking, so the call often comes during the morning surgery.

A history should be obtained from the patient, or from the relatives if there are speech difficulties. A sudden onset of symptoms in a patient with risk factors makes the diagnosis secure. If the history is not typical, there may be an underlying progressive process which needs to be identified and treated.

Stroke is by a long way the commonest reason for the sudden onset of a neurological deficit in an elderly person. Other possibilities should also be borne in mind. A gradual onset of symptoms over hours or days will suggest a non-stroke lesion such as subdural haematoma, cerebral tumour or cerebral abscess. An abrupt onset of symptoms followed by a rapid deterioration but no focal neurological signs can be due to a cerebellar stroke complicated by acute obstructive hydrocephalus, or by a large intracranial haemorrhage.

Having confirmed a diagnosis of stroke, the neurological symptoms will be getting worse, getting better or will be stable.

1. Symptoms getting worse. This may be a stroke in evolution or an intacranial bleed. Hospital admission is urgent.
2. Symptoms getting better. The patient may be having a TIA. A further visit later in the day or the next day will clarify the picture.
3. Symptoms stable. If the overall clinical condition does not warrant admission, it is useful to wait for a few hours or a day to see if there will be an improvement in symptoms.

What examination is useful?

Neurological signs

An early assessment of the degree of neurological impairment will give an indication of the likely prognosis as the more severe the stroke, the less likely is good recovery.

Haemorrhagic or ischaemic?
The distinction between whether a bleeding event or a clotting event has caused the stroke cannot be made on clinical grounds alone.[1] This is, however, a distinction of some importance as the death rate following haemorrhagic stroke is higher, and the usual secondary preventive strategies for ischaemic stroke may make haemorrhagic stroke worse.

Eighty per cent of strokes are caused by ischaemia and 20% by haemorrhage. Computed tomography (CT) scan is the best way of checking which is which. It has to be done in the first 14 days after a stroke or the typical appearance will have resolved.[1]

Where has the stroke occurred?
Detecting the probable site of the lesion can be of professional interest as well as predicting the likely disabilities to come.

Ninety per cent of strokes affect the cerebral hemispheres, and of these 75% occur in the territory of the internal carotid artery and 15% in the vertebrobasilar artery territory (in the other 10% the picture is not clear).[2]

Carotid territory strokes cause hemiparesis and facial paresis, monocular visual loss, dysarthria, dysphasia (dysphasia of language if the dominant hemisphere is involved, or visuospatial dysphasia if the non-dominant hemisphere is involved), conjugate gaze to the side of the lesion, and homonymous hemianopia.

Vertebrobasilar territory strokes cause bilateral blindness, homonymous hemianopia, diplopia and nystagmus, problems with gait and stance, vertigo, hemi- or bilateral motor paresis, hemi- or bilateral sensory loss and dysarthria.

Heart sounds

Clinical evidence of a valvular lesion, or a finding of atrial fibrillation either with or without a valve lesion will indicate that anticoagulation should be considered.[7]

Blood pressure

Blood pressure rises acutely with a stroke, and then spontaneously falls over the next few days.[1] A few days after the stroke more representative readings can be obtained. A decision whether or not to treat hypertension should be delayed until at least 10 days after the stroke.[8]

A low blood pressure may suggest the rare instance of a stroke brought on by haemodynamic problems where the amount of blood perfusing the brain is reduced, leading to neurological deficit.

Bruits

A bruit over the carotid artery should be listened for. Its presence indicates vascular pathology, but does not indicate the degree of any carotid stenosis[5] since tight stenosis does not let enough blood through to cause a bruit.

What about investigations?

Investigations are suggested routinely to detect other remediable underlying pathology. These might include full blood count, erythrocyte sedimentation rate, blood glucose, urea and electrolytes, serum cholesterol, chest X-ray and electrocardiogram. These will help to detect any underlying treatable conditions such as haematological disorders, cerebral arteritis, bacterial endocarditis, diabetes mellitus, ischaemic heart disease, atrial fibrillation and other cardiac disorders.

Does the patient need acute admission?

If the patient clearly needs admitting, then the only requirement is to confirm the diagnosis and alert the hospital to any relevant past history. If it is intended that the patient be kept at home, then an underlying cause for the stroke which may benefit from hospitalization should be ruled out.

The following clinical features may indicate that the diagnosis is not a stroke, or that specialist care will be beneficial:[9]

- Diagnostic doubt.
- Headache.
- Dysphagia. This occurs after a third of strokes.[1]
- Presence of potential complicating factors such as severe hypertension or type I diabetes.
- Impaired consciousness.
- Fever.
- Youth – patient under 45 years.
- Presence of treatable risk factors such as valvular heart disease.
- Absence of obvious risk factors.
- Neck stiffness; positive Kernig's sign.
- Evidence of raised intracranial pressure.

Will the patient benefit from later admission?

If there is no immediate indication for admission, and the carers and patient can contain the situation for a few hours or overnight, a much clearer decision can be made about whether the patient would benefit from admission.

About 80% of stroke victims are admitted to hospital,[10] but this varies in different parts of the country so that in some areas around half of cases are kept at home.

1. There is no treatment modality which is known to reduce the neurological damage following a stroke.[3] However, organized stroke care (with the emphasis on organized) may reduce short- and long-term mortality by about 25%, and reduce the longer-term disability at least over the first 6 months.[11] If a proper stroke unit is available, there is little justification in denying the stroke victim access to the facilities. On the other hand, if the stroke is so severe that death is imminent and there is good family support, little can be gained by admission.
2. The only way of determining which are the 20% of strokes

which are haemorrhagic and hence in which antithrombotic treatment should not be used is by CT scan, which is only available in the hospital setting.
3. Some patients are so severely affected that intensive nursing support is needed.

Most patients who would benefit from specialist care will need admission, but in some it may be possible for them to receive any necessary treatment through the outpatient clinic.

What happens after a stroke? Answering the patient's questions

The outlook after a stroke is not very good. Patients and their carers are entitled to accurate information, however distressing this may be. Creating unrealistic expectations causes more problems in the long run.

Death

The patient suffering a stroke will have a 20% chance of dying within the first month after it.[1] Of these deaths, half will be due to the acute effects of the stroke, and half due to complications, for example pneumonia.

Ten years later the patient has under a 50% chance of still being alive. Fifteen per cent will suffer a subsequent fatal stroke, but 40% will die of a myocardial infarction.[12] Stroke is only one manifestation of vascular disease.

Disability

Eighty per cent of stroke victims live in the community, but 25% are entirely dependent on a carer, and a further 30% need help with daily living tasks. Hence fewer than half of all stroke victims end up being fully independent.[13]

After 6 months, 50–80% of patients will be able to walk, but only 22% can walk at their previous speed.[14]

Around 25% of stroke sufferers become depressed.[15] This is about twice the level of the normal elderly population (at 15%), and is about the same as for other elderly people with a chronic debilitating illness. The site and extent of the cerebral damage does not correlate well with the chance of depression.

Recurrence

After a stroke, the victim has a 13% chance of recurrence in the first year, and 5% per year thereafter.[3]

What to do after the stroke

Patients kept at home should have their rehabilitation begun at once (provided they are fit enough). The physiotherapist should be involved at an early stage to prevent contractures and encourage and plan mobilization. Occupational therapy involvement will concentrate on the assessment of tasks of daily living, aids, adaptations to the home, and support for carers. District nursing input may be needed for those with major nursing needs.

The stroke patient who is admitted to hospital will usually be discharged after an average of 2–3 weeks, during which time there should have been an intensive rehabilitative effort. It is important that discharge be properly planned so that community support structures can be set up. Close liaison between hospital and primary care in all disciplines is vital.

Secondary prevention

The risk of death after a first stroke is significantly raised. If a stroke has occurred, it means that there exists significant vascular pathology. The risk of subsequent death through a heart attack is greater than that of death from a further stroke.

Risk factors should be attended to where appropriate (see later for a discussion of risk factors). Patients with the greatest risk levels have the most to gain from preventive measures.

Hypertension
Hypertension should be brought under control gradually. The blood pressure levels at which treatment will be beneficial are lower than for the treatment of hypertension without end-organ damage. Either a systolic pressure over 160 mmHg or a diastolic above 90 mmHg is probably worth treatment.

Elderly patients are at greater stroke risk, and so potentially have more to gain from treatment. Treating hypertension in the very old has yet to demonstrate benefit conclusively, but there is clear advantage to be gained up to age 80.[16]

Lifestyle
Smoking should be counselled against. A low-fat diet is reasonable advice, though the protective value of cholesterol-lowering drugs is unsure.[1]

What about aspirin?
Following a stroke, the risk of a future serious vascular event (further stroke, heart attack or death from vascular causes) can be reduced by about 25% by treatment with aspirin.[17] The benefit is only seen in patients who have had an ischaemic stroke, and though there is an 80% chance that any given stroke will be ischaemic, the diagnosis can only be made definitively after CT scan. Following haemorrhagic stroke, aspirin should not be used.

Doses between 150 and 300 mg/day seem effective, and doses as low as 37.5 mg are beneficial if higher doses cause gastric irritation.[1] The effects of the aspirin on platelet stickiness only last about 3 days, and an acute vascular event may reduce this time substantially, so that daily doses of aspirin are preferable to alternate days.[18]

Benefits from continuing aspirin treatment up to 2 years after a stroke have been demonstrated. It is probable that the benefits will continue and so indefinite use of aspirin is recommended.[17]

Anticoagulation
The place of anticoagulation in the secondary prevention of stroke is unclear. Patients with atrial fibrillation and a probable cardiac source of emboli will benefit.[1]

Rehabilitation – tertiary prevention

In the early weeks the treatment of the stroke victim is usually very intensive, and such intensity has been shown to be of some benefit. However, it is not clear which of the types of intervention work and which do not; it is only known that the totality is of benefit.

In the early days after a stroke there is usually an intense rehabilitative effort. On discharge from hospital, this intensity is much reduced, which can lead to a sense of rejection. At this stage the GP assumes responsibility and the community team has to be mobilized.

It is suggested that recovery from a stroke goes through four stages:[19] crisis, treatment, realization and adjustment. Hospitals tend to concentrate on the first two. This can lead patients and carers to believe that this is the only form of treatment available. Despondency results when it is evident that a degree of disability will persist.

Intrinsic recovery, that is the return of neurological function, occurs over the first 3 months only.

Functional recovery, that is the ability to do things, occurs by a combination of intrinsic recovery and adaptation. The full process may take up to 12 months, with 5–10% of the improvement happening in the latter 6 months. Further improvement after 12 months is very unlikely.[14]

Despite this, in one study 65% of spouses were still expecting the full recovery of the patient 16 months after the stroke.[13] There is a need for realistic information and explanation so that other ways of minimizing disability can be looked for at an early stage.

The role of the GP in stroke rehabilitation

Accessibility

One study found that at 3 months after discharge one-third of stroke victims had still not seen their GP.[10] In the same study, 27% had had no inpatient physiotherapy, and 67% no outpatient physiotherapy. An early assessment should be made, and community services mobilized if this has not already been done.

The GP also has a *gatekeeper role* to provide the patient with access to other services.

Information

Informed and realistic information and advice are needed by the patient and carers. This can be supplemented by the excellent literature available from the Stroke Association CHSA House, Whitecross Street, London EC1Y 8JJ. Tel. 0171 490 7999 (previously part of the Heart, Chest and Stroke Association).

A discussion of prognosis is appropriate. Advice on resumption of normal activities can be useful, especially with relation to sexual activity – only a third of patients return to their previous levels of sexual activity after a stroke.[14] Advice on eating, smoking and alcohol may be needed.

Secondary prevention

See the earlier discussion.

Symptom control

Depression

Depression is very common among stroke victims. It should be specifically looked for as it will respond to antidepressants in standard doses (75–150 mg of tricyclic a day). Bear in mind that the average stroke victim will be elderly and the stroke indicates that there is significant vascular pathology. If urinary retention or cardiac arrhythmia is likely, then the newer antidepressants with fewer side-effects can be useful. Elderly patients will anyway tend to respond to lower dosages of antidepressant medication.

Depression should be distinguished from *emotionalism* which also frequently accompanies a stroke. Patients may become weepy and distressed for no obvious reason, to their embarrassment and the distress of their carers. Emotionalism may show some response to antidepressants. In general, management should include steps to make sure that carers are not reinforcing this particular type of illness behaviour.

Pain

Pain, in particular shoulder pain, may be present. Spastic muscles are prone to spasm. Muscle and even bone injuries may occur. Pressure areas need regular review. Pain may respond to simple analgesia such as paracetamol 1000 mg 6-hourly, or aspirin 300–900 mg 4-hourly if there is an inflammatory element to the pain and there are no contraindications.

In addition, stroke sufferers are subject to *central poststroke pain* (CPSP or thalamic syndrome). This affects between 2 and 6% of victims and is commoner in the younger patient.[20] Symptoms do not usually appear immediately after the stroke, and are usually delayed several weeks or months. An area of burning pain is felt, often associated with autonomic instability and allodynia (the feeling of pain following non-painful stimuli). There is invariably an area of sensory loss to pinprick which extends beyond the bounds of the pain.

CPSP is not nociceptive pain and so usual analgesics do not work. Nortriptyline and amitriptyline in standard doses (75–150 mg/day) will help, but they do not have a licence for use in pain relief. Response takes 4–6 weeks.

Insomnia and incontinence

Insomnia and incontinence may not be volunteered unless enquired after.

Leg swelling and contractures
Leg swelling and contractures in the affected limbs will be visible on clinical examination.

Pressure sores and fractures
Pressure sores and fractures are commoner in the stroke victim.

Psychological support

Problems of psychological adaptation will be present to a greater or lesser extent in all stroke survivors.

Communication difficulty either with speech or language will benefit from involvement with a speech therapist.

Impaired mobility may benefit from aids and adaptations, and modified transport. The Driver and Vehicle Licensing Authority (DVLA) should be notified after a stroke and *driving* counselled against for at least the first month.[4] After this it may be possible to restart, but epilepsy and hemianopia are obvious barriers. A less obvious problem is sensory inattention. If the DVLA is in doubt, an independent medical and a formal test of driving ability will be organized.

Dependence and boredom are almost universal among stroke victims. Very few patients readily adapt their hobbies to their disabilities and will tend to dwell on what they cannot do rather than on what they can do. These attitudes need to be identified and counselled against.

Dealing with crises

The two major crisis points are at the time of the stroke, and on discharge from hospital. The withdrawal of active therapy may give a sense of rejection. If the carer becomes ill or dies, or there is an additional health problem such as a fracture, then the whole care plan has to be rethought.

Supporting the carer

Most of the care of stroke victims in the community is done by informal carers. The majority of these are spouses, and so usually elderly themselves. Next in order of frequency are daughters and daughters-in-law. Fourteen per cent of carers will have given up work to look after the stroke victim.[13]

Around 12% of stroke carers are depressed, and this figure is 40% in the case of spouses.[13] The patient's wife is thus more likely to be depressed than the patient.

Financial advice
Financial advice is often needed. Some benefits are particularly relevant to the stroke victim, such as the Attendance Allowance and Disability Living Allowance. Further advice can be obtained via advice centres or social workers.

Respite admissions and day care can give the carer a well-earned rest.

The Stroke Association, other voluntary bodies and many hospital stroke units provide Stroke Clubs for the support of patient and carer, but these facilities are often not known about.

Primary prevention

Following the 1990 GP contract, a lot of effort is going into opportunistic and population screening for vascular disorders. The arguments for and against these efforts are well-rehearsed.

As far as stroke is concerned, the routine use of aspirin for primary prevention is not recommended.[18] In the person at low risk of a stroke, the benefits are very small and so the unacceptability of gastric side-effects is correspondingly greater.

If atrial fibrillation of non-valvular cause is found in an asymptomatic patient, the risk of stroke increases fivefold, and atrial fibrillation is present in 15% of patients who have had a stroke.[7] Warfarin treatment to keep the international normalized ratio (INR) between 1.5 and 3 reduces the risk of first-time strokes by two-thirds.[7] In practice, a large part of the potential recipients of warfarin for this indication will have a contraindication – the exclusions from many of the trials which produced evidence of benefit were very large.

The population approach to prevention

The *Health of the Nation* has suggested targets for primary prevention of stroke:[10]

- To reduce the death rate for stroke in people under the age of 65 years by at least 40% by the year 2000 (from 12.5/100 000 in 1990 to no more than 7.5/100 000).
- To reduce the death rate from stroke in people aged 65–74 years by at least 40% by the year 2000 (from 265/100 000 in 1990 to no more than 159/100 000).

These targets have implications for other aspects of government policy as well as for the health service. A major risk factor for stroke is raised blood pressure. It is estimated that a reduction of 50 mmol/l in the average amount of salt ingested would lower the average diastolic blood pressure by 5 mmHg, and this would lead to a reduction in mortality from stroke of 22%.[3] This could be achieved by reducing the salt used in food processing.

Changes in the labelling of processed foods, further restrictions on cigarette advertising and the reduction of alcohol and cigarette consumption through increasing prices could bring about substantial improvements in the incidence of stroke.[3]

The individual approach to prevention

The at-risk factors for stroke are identical to those for coronary heart disease. Hypertension seems to be of more significance and cholesterol of less significance than for coronary heart disease. An opportunistic approach to risk assessment is recommended.[10]

What are the risk factors for stroke?

Eighty per cent of stroke victims have one or more risk factor.[2]

Previous cerebrovascular episode

After a stroke, the victim has a 13% chance of recurrence in the first year, and 5% per year thereafter.[3]

Smoking

Smoking increases the risk of a first stroke by 50%.[3]

Hypertension

Fifty per cent of victims of first stroke have raised blood pressure.[2]

Ischaemic heart disease

Coronary heart disease is found in 40% of stroke victims.[2]

Diabetes

Around 10% of first stroke victims have diabetes mellitus.[2]

Social factors

The mortality rate from stroke varies with area of the country, and with social class. For instance, the death rate in Scotland is 50% higher than in West Thames. In men from 20 to 64, the standardized mortality ratio in social class 1 is 62 compared with 179 in social class 5.[10] If the mortality rates could all be brought down to those of the lowest geographical area and social class, substantial overall improvements would result.

Transient ischaemic attack

A TIA is the same as a stroke in all respects of definition, except that the symptoms resolve completely within 24 hours. Amaurosis fugax is a transient monocular visual loss lasting under 24 hours (and usually a couple of minutes only). This and TIA are due to small emboli which, in 75% of cases, arise from the internal carotid artery.[2]

There are 25 000 TIAs a year in the UK – an incidence of 1 per 1000, or 2 per average GP list. Having a TIA increases the risk of a subsequent stroke in the next year 13-fold,[5] and 15% of all strokes are preceded by TIA.[2]

The internal carotid artery may reveal a bruit, but in 30–50% of cases this is not present either because the stenosis is too great or too little. The degree of stenosis can only be finally determined by angiography, a procedure which carries a 1–2% chance of causing a stroke.[1] Suitable candidates for angiography can be detected by prior use of carotid ultrasound.

The diagnosis of TIA may be difficult as there are many other reasons why patients have dizzy spells. In one series only a third of patients referred to a clinic with a diagnosis of TIA had been correctly diagnosed.[2]

Carotid endarterectomy will benefit patients who have degrees of stenosis above 70%.[5] There is a 4–5% risk of stroke with the operation, but the subsequent stroke risk is returned to average levels.[1]

References

1. Sandercock PA and Lindley RI. Management of acute stroke. *Prescribers' J* 1993; **33**: 196–205
2. Naylor AR and Bell PRF. Management of mild symptomatic CVD. *Update* 1993; **47**: 670–5

3. Dennis M and Warlow C. Strategy for stroke. *Br Med J* 1991; **303**: 636–8
4. Driving after a stroke or TIA. The Stroke Association Leaflet 5. 1994
5. Naylor AR. Carotid endarterectomy for the prevention of ischaemic stroke. The Stroke Association Leaflet 2. 1993
6. Greveson G and James O. Improving long-term outcome after stroke – the views of carers. *Health Trends* 1991; **23**: 1612
7. Lowe GDO. Antithrombotic treatment and atrial fibrillation. *Br Med J* 1992; **305**: 1445–6
8. O'Connell JE and Gray CS. Treating hypertension after stroke. *Br Med J* 1994; **308**: 1523–4
9. Lees K and Reid J. Stroke. *The Practitioner* 1991; **235**: 570–4
10. Crowe S. Stroke prevention: more than just monitoring BP. *Monitor Weekly* 1993; **6**: 41–2
11. Sandercock P. Managing stroke: the way forward. *Br Med J* 1993; **307**: 1297–8
12. Marshall J. Why patients at risk of stroke should take aspirin. *Monitor Weekly* 1994; **7**: 43–4
13. Cassidy TP and Gray CS. Stroke and the carer. *Br J Gen Pract* 1991; **41**: 267–8
14. Hewer RL. Stroke-induced disability. *Update* 1994; **48**: 375–85
15. House A. Depression after stroke. *Br Med J* 1987; **294**: 76–8
16. Sever P, Beevers G, Bulpitt C *et al.* Management guidelines in essential hypertension: report of the second working party of the British Hypertension Society. *Br Med J* 1993; **306**: 983–7
17. Underwood MJ and More RS. The aspirin papers. *Br Med J* 1994; **308**: 71–2
18. Aspirin to prevent heart attack or stroke. *Drug Ther Bull* 1994; **32**: 71–2
19. Forster A and Young J. Stroke rehabilitation: can we do better? *Br Med J* 1992; **305**: 1446–7
20. Bowsher D. Central post-stroke pain and its treatment. The Stroke Association Leaflet 3

4

Heart failure

Aims

The trainee should:

- Have knowledge of the symptoms and signs of heart failure.
- Be able to institute appropriate therapy in acute and chronic heart failure.
- Know which patients with heart failure would benefit from referral.

Who gets heart failure?

Figures from the Framingham study show that the incidence of new cases of chronic heart failure doubles with each decade of age from 45 years:[1]

Under 65 years	1%
65–74 years	3%
Over 75 years	10%
Over 85 years	20%

In the overwhelming majority of sufferers in the UK the underlying cause is ischaemic heart disease (IHD).[2] The risk factors are therefore those for IHD, notably smoking, obesity, raised cholesterol, hypertension, diabetes, male sex, family history and getting older. The increasing number of elderly people will increase the number of sufferers.

Why is heart failure important?

Heart failure, in its severe forms, carries a mortality rate far higher than most cancers.[2] The New York Heart Association[11] has defined four grades of heart failure, a classification which is now used worldwide:

Class I: No limitation of ordinary physical activity and no symptoms on ordinary activity; 5-year mortality 10–20%.[1]

Class II: Slight limitation of physical activity, symptoms on ordinary activity such as walking uphill or climbing stairs but comfortable at rest; 5-year mortality 10–20%.

Class III: Marked limitation of physical activity. Symptoms present on less than ordinary activity, such as walking on the flat ground, but still comfortable at rest; 5-year mortality 50–70%.

Class IV: Any physical activity causes discomfort. Symptoms are present at rest; 5-year mortality 70–100%.

In addition to this mortality, heart failure causes significant morbidity. When compared with other chronic debilitating illnesses such as diabetes, arthritis and hypertension, heart failure has been shown in surveys to cause a significantly greater negative impact on the quality of life.[2] Each year in the UK there are 120 000 hospital admissions for heart failure, which is 5% of all adult medical and geriatric admissions. The total NHS bill is about £360m. a year (1993 prices), of which 60% is spent on hospital care.

Why does heart failure happen?

Heart failure occurs when the heart is unable to pump blood around quickly enough to sustain normal levels of activity. The failure can be further divided according to the part of the heart primarily involved – left heart failure, right heart failure and biventricular failure. Failure of the left ventricle is the commonest cause of heart failure. In practical terms, however, failure of either the left or right ventricles rapidly spreads to involve the whole circulation, meaning that heart failure can be treated as a single entity.

If either the pumping ability of the heart is reduced, or the work required of the heart is increased, the effect is the same.

- Reduced pumping ability occurs if the myocardium is damaged, valve function is impaired, or the heart becomes stiff so that insufficient blood is admitted to the heart during diastole. Causes include ischaemia/infarction, valvular disease, cardiomyopathies, congenital heart disease, myocarditis, alcoholic cardiomyopathy and atrial myxoma.[1]

● Increased heart work occurs if there is an increased resistance in the circulation – the so-called cardiac afterload. Typical causes include aortic and pulmonary stenosis, hypertension and coarctation of the aorta.[1]

When there is reduced cardiac output, compensatory mechanisms come into play. Unfortunately, these mechanisms readily become overwhelmed, and the heart failure becomes decompensated.

1. Reduced cardiac output reduces renal perfusion. This stimulates the increase of renin, angiotensinogen, angiotensin I and, via angiotensin-converting enzyme (ACE), angiotensin II. Angiotensin II increases sympathetic drive and vasoconstriction, and causes more aldosterone to be produced which increases sodium and water retention and thus increases blood volume.[3]

2. Reduced cardiac output also leads to a fall in blood pressure, and this activates the sympathetic nervous system. This increases both the heart rate and the peripheral resistance of the circulation.

The increase in blood volume and decrease in the vascular bed is designed to compensate for the reduced cardiac output. However, this is also the process that leads to the symptoms of heart failure. Treatment therefore attempts to override the body's own compensatory mechanisms.

How is heart failure recognized clinically?

In the later stages of heart failure there are clinical signs and making the diagnosis is not a problem. Early stages of heart failure are diagnosed when a patient with known or suspected heart disease presents with fatigue, lethargy and tiredness. These are non-specific symptoms, and at this stage of the disease the GP can only expect to diagnose about 50% of cases correctly.[4]

Symptoms

● Breathlessness.
● Fatigue.
● Oedema.

Signs

- Pulmonary or peripheral oedema.
- Tachycardia.
- A third heart sound, with or without a gallop rhythm.
- Cardiomegaly.

What investigations are useful?

Echocardiography

This is the most useful investigation in heart failure.[2] Any reversible causes of the failure such as valve or pericardial disease can be readily identified. The usual finding, however, is of a poorly contracting left ventricle. Unfortunately echocardiography is not generally available to GPs on an open access basis.

Chest X-ray

The chest X-ray in heart failure will often show cardiomegaly, and may be helpful in diagnosing pulmonary oedema if there is some clinical doubt.

Electrocardiogram

The electrocardiogram in heart failure is rarely normal.[2] There may be the pathological Q waves of a previous myocardial infarction, and left ventricular hypertrophy or an arrhythmia may be detected.

Treating acute heart failure

In acute heart failure, there is a sudden onset of breathlessness associated with bilateral basal crepitations. Left heart failure usually predominates, but there may be right heart failure as well, leading to a raised jugulovenous pressure. Whether this acute episode is a new event or occurs against a background of known cardiac pathology does not matter as far as immediate treatment is concerned.

The patient should be sat up in bed, and oxygen given if available. Intravenous loop diuretics such as 40 mg frusemide or 1 mg bumetanide are required. Intravenous diamorphine 2.5–5 mg or morphine 5–10 mg will relieve pulmonary oedema and anxiety.[3]

Bear in mind that the elderly and those with chronic pulmonary disease may be particularly susceptible to the respiratory-depressant side-effects of opiates, and so smaller doses should be used, at least in the first instance. Urgent transfer to hospital is needed.[5]

Treating chronic heart failure

Is there a reversible cause?

The electrocardiogram and chest X-ray and the echocardiogram (if available) will give some indication whether the heart failure has a remediable cause, or a remediable component. In some patients there may be compensated heart failure which has been either under control or symptomless, but which then begins to cause trouble. There may have been a myocardial infarction which has caused the emergence of symptoms, but there are other possibilities:

* Infection, especially of the chest.
* Bacterial endocarditis.
* Drugs such as non-steroidal anti-inflammatory drugs (NSAIDs), steroids, calcium channel blockers, β-blockers, thyroxine in overdosage, lithium, antacids with a high sodium content, and some antiarrhythmic drugs.
* Anaemia.
* Thyrotoxicosis.
* Arrhythmias such as fast atrial fibrillation and the brady-arrhythmias.

Diuretics

Diuretics are the most effective symptomatic remedy for heart failure,[2] and so are the first line of treatment in all degrees of severity.

Loop diuretics such as frusemide can be used at a dose of 40 mg/day. This is the most effective dose, but in some patients reduced efficacy is seen and so doses up to 120 mg/day are needed. The diuresis produced is quite brisk but lasts only around 6 hours. So that sleep is not disturbed, it is usual to take the entire dose shortly after waking. In some instances, however, where paroxysmal nocturnal dyspnoea is a particular problem, part or all of the dose can be given later in the day so that excess fluid is cleared out before sleep is attempted.

Thiazides such as bendrofluazide have a ceiling of effect at around 10 mg,[6] and act over the full 24 hours. They are less powerful than the loop diuretics.

Sometimes a thiazide can usefully be used in conjunction with a loop diuretic, as they work on different parts of the nephron. This improves diuresis, but careful monitoring of hydration status and blood chemistry is required, usually necessitating inpatient supervision.[2]

When using diuretics, it is important to have regard to body potassium levels, and in particular hypokalaemia. Hypokalaemia itself may produce symptoms such as tiredness and lethargy, and may also precipitate arrhythmias which will aggravate the heart failure. Serum potassium should be measured before treatment and after 3 months of treatment. It is the level of intracellular potassium which is important, and though serum levels do not necessarily correlate closely with this, a serum sample is easy to obtain and acts as a useful proxy measure.

If the level of serum potassium falls below 3.0 mmol/l, then this may represent clinically significant hypokalaemia.[5] The concomitant use of a potassium-sparing diuretic such as amiloride 5 mg a day is recommended.

Angiotensin-converting enzyme inhibitors

These drugs have substantially altered the management of heart failure. The CONSENSUS study[7] on patients with severe (class IV) heart failure showed that the use of enalapril reduced the 6-month and 1-year chance of death by 40 and 31% respectively. Later trials have shown that the use of ACE inhibitors with diuretics improves the symptoms and prognosis in all grades of heart failure.[2] Since heart failure has such an awful prognosis untreated, ACE inhibitors have a considerable impact on overall mortality rates in heart failure sufferers. Even if the symptoms can be completely relieved by diuretics, there is still a strong case for adding an ACE inhibitor to improve prognosis.

Putting this in perspective, in severe heart failure, treating 1000 patients for a year with enalapril will prevent 160 deaths. In moderate heart failure, 16 deaths and 116 hospital admissions are avoided. Compare this with the 1–2 strokes per year prevented by treating 1000 mild hypertensives, and the 25 deaths prevented from treating 1000 myocardial infarctions with streptokinase.[8]

The major trials have been done using enalapril, but it is likely that the other members of the group have similar effects.

ACE inhibitors reduce the production of angiotensin II, which is responsible for vasoconstrictor and some renal effects. In addition, they increase the concentration of the vasodilator bradykinin, and have effects on the kidneys, electrolytes and the electrical stability of the heart.[2]

How should an ACE inhibitor be started?

At home or in hospital? When an ACE inhibitor is started, the first dose may cause significant hypotension. In the early days of their use, this led to the recommendation that the drugs should only be commenced under inpatient guidance. This fear has proved to be exaggerated, and now captopril, enalapril and lisinopril all have licences allowing their initiation in primary care.[3]

In addition, ACE inhibitors tend to raise serum potassium levels. This is useful when they are used together with a diuretic as the effects on potassium tend to cancel each other out. If potassium supplements or potassium-sparing drugs are being used, however, this can lead to troublesome hyperkalaemia.

Some groups are at particular risk of an unpleasant reaction, and for them it is still recommended that any ACE inhibitor should be started as an inpatient:[3]

- Severe heart failure.
- High-dose diuretics, more than 80 mg frusemide or equivalent.
- Patients with hypovolaemia.
- Patients with hyponatraemia (plasma sodium under 130 mmol/l).
- Pre-existing hypotension (systolic pressure under 90 mmHg).
- Unstable heart failure.
- Renal impairment (plasma creatinine above 150 μmol/l).
- Receiving high-dose vasodilator therapy.
- Aged 70 or over.

Monitoring treatment

1. *Before treatment:* stop any potassium supplements and potassium-sparing diuretics.
2. *The day before starting treatment:* stop other diuretics.
3. *The starting day:* the patient should be lying or sitting, and a small dose of treatment taken (e.g. enalapril 2.5 mg or captopril 6.25 mg). The patient should be asked to stay sitting or lying for the next 4 hours.
4. *The next day:* the diuretics can be restarted. Potassium supplements and potassium-sparing diuretics should not be restarted as ACE inhibitors have a potassium-sparing effect, and hyperkalaemia may result. The dose of ACE inhibitor should

rise to 2.5 mg enalapril twice a day, 12.5 mg captopril thrice a day, or equivalent.
5. *After 2 weeks:* check the urea and electrolytes. As long as the serum potassium is under 5 mmol/l, the serum creatinine is less than 200 μmol/l and there are no symptoms of hypotension, the ACE inhibitor dose can be raised to the higher levels which are known to convey the most benefit,[2] notably enalapril 10 mg twice a day or captopril 25–50 mg thrice a day.

Haemodynamic improvement can be detected quite quickly, but clinical improvement may take 4–6 weeks to appear.[6]

Some 5–10% of patients taking ACE inhibitors develop a dry cough. Heart failure also causes cough in around 30% of cases, and in none of the trials has cough been a significant cause of drop-out.[2]

There are potentially serious interactions between ACE inhibitors and NSAIDs (renal impairment) and lithium (lithium toxicity).

Digoxin

At one time, digoxin was widely used as a treatment for heart failure as it has inotropic and antiarrhythmic properties. Then its popularity declined as it was felt only to be useful where atrial fibrillation coexisted. The evidence has been re-evaluated, and digoxin is now known to be of benefit in patients with heart failure who are in sinus rhythm.[2] The benefit is not as great as with diuretics and ACE inhibitors, but there is an added effect. Digoxin is thus recommended when symptoms persist despite full diuretic and ACE inhibitor therapy, or with diuretics if an ACE inhibitor cannot be tolerated.

Digoxin toxicity is a relatively rare event, but is more likely in the presence of hypokalaemia. ACE inhibitors slightly raise serum potassium, and diuretics lower it. It is not appropriate to be obsessive about potassium levels as serum potassium bears little relation to intracellular potassium levels. However, it is wise to check levels after a month on a new treatment, and institute replacement if hypokalaemia has occurred.

There is an interaction with quinine, a treatment often used in the types of patient who have heart failure, and with amiodarone. If either of these is prescribed, the dose of digoxin should be halved.[9]

Between 10 and 50% of patients with heart failure will also be in atrial fibrillation anyway,[2] making the benefits of digoxin even more attractive. For a discussion of the use of anticoagulation in patients with atrial fibrillation in order to prevent cerebrovascular events, please see Chapter 3.

Other treatments

Vasodilators such as nitrates and hydralazine have been shown to improve the symptoms and exercise tolerance in severe degrees of heart failure, but not as much as ACE inhibitors. Whether there is an improvement in mortality is not firmly established.[2]

Non-drug treatments

Weight reduction should be encouraged in the obese. Cigarette smoking and over indulgence in alcohol should be discouraged. Fluid restriction is usually unnecessary except in severe cases which are proving difficult to bring under control. Rest in bed is important in acute left ventricular failure, but in chronic heart failure a graded exercise programme has been shown to improve exercise tolerance.[10]

The psychological impact of heart failure can be considerable. The limitations on function and the adverse effects on quality of life are often severe. Even the phrase heart failure is a particularly poignant reminder of the possible seriousness of the condition. It is impossible to be too optimistic about the eventual prognosis in a patient with heart failure. It should be possible to relieve the symptoms, however.

As with all chronic debilitating diseases, sufferers may react in a variety of ways:

- Some patients will deny the existence of the problem and not cooperate with treatment.
- Some patients will be devastated by the diagnosis and so withdraw from all their usual activities. As the excessive rest deconditions their body, even low levels of exertion will lead to breathlessness and fatigue. This will reinforce the serious and progressive nature of the disease. Depression and dependence are common.
- Other sufferers will become 'professional patients'. Their whole life will become geared round medication and other modes of therapy, again to the exclusion of all else. Compliance will usually be exemplary, and any changes in symptoms will undoubtedly be reported without delay. Living with such a patient can be a trying experience.
- Probably the best response to the diagnosis is an optimistic resignation. There will be limitations of function, but some tasks can be achieved more slowly, and others by altering how they are tackled. New interests and hobbies which take account of the

patient's limitations are to be encouraged. Appropriate treatments can be recommended both because they help the symptoms, and because they help the patient live longer.

Which patients might benefit from referral?

- If a remediable cause for the heart failure is found or suspected.
- If cardiac surgery might be helpful (valve disease, coronary artery bypass).
- If an echocardiogram is desirable and cannot otherwise be arranged.
- If symptoms persist despite the full measure of the treatments with which the GP feels comfortable.

References

1. Kassianos G. Chronic heart failure. *Care Elderly* 1993; **5**: 298–9
2. Dargie HJ and McMurray JJV. Diagnosis and management of heart failure. *Br Med J* 1994; **308**: 321–8
3. ACE inhibitors in the treatment of heart failure. *MeReC Bull* 1994; **5**: 1–4
4. Wheeldon N, MacDonald T and Flucker CJ *et al*. Chronic heart failure in the community: an echocardiographic study of its prevalence and an assessment of the workload it generates for primary health care and hospital physicians. *Q J Medi* 1993; **86**: 17–23
5. Managing heart failure – home or hospital? *Drug Ther Bull* 1992; **30**: 61–63
6. Waller D. Chronic cardiac failure. *Prescribers' J* 1992; **32**: 185–92
7. CONSENSUS Trial Study Group. Effects of enalapril on mortality in severe congestive heart failure. Results of the co-operative Scandinavian enalapril survival study. *N Engl J Med* 1987; **816**: 142–935
8. McMurray J and Dargie HJ. Coronary heart disease. *Br Med J* 1991; **303**: 1546–7
9. *British National Formulary* 27. London: British Medical Association/Royal Pharmaceutical Society of Great Britain 1994
10. Taskforce Working Group on Cardiac Rehabilitation of the European Society of Cardiology. Chronic heart failure. *Eur Heart J* 1992; **13**(suppl): 42–4
11. Criteria Committee, New York Heart Association Inc. Disease of the heart and blood vessels. Nomenclature and Criteria for Diagnoses, 6th ed. Boston: Little Brown & Co. 1992 p 214

5

Depression

Aims

The trainee should:

- Be able to conduct a consultation which makes a diagnosis of depression more likely.
- Be aware of the interventions available within general practice.
- Be able to construct a care plan for a depressed patient.

What is depression?

Depressive illness can usefully be divided into major depression and then everything else. This is a distinction of some importance as the following definition of major depression is used in trials of treatment. The definition defines an illness, and also predicts the likely response to treatment.

Major depression

The definition of major depression most widely used is that taken from the revised third edition of the *Diagnostic and Statistical Manual* of the American Psychiatric Association (*DSM-III-R*).[1] This may be summarized as at least five of the following symptoms present during the same 2-week period. This must include at least one of the symptoms of depressed mood or diminished interest or pleasure.

- Depressed mood.
- Markedly diminished interest or pleasure in normal activities.
- Significant weight gain or loss.
- Insomnia or hypersomnia.
- Being agitated or retarded.
- Fatigue or loss of energy.

- Feelings of worthlessness or excessive guilt.
- Diminished ability to think or concentrate, or indecisiveness.
- Recurrent thoughts of death or suicidal thoughts/actions.

Sleep in the depressed patient is usually reduced. Early waking is particularly significant. Some, especially the young, have hypersomnia – the Dormouse Syndrome.

Other depressions

Other milder depressive syndromes are often found in general practice:[2]

1. Depressive episodes that do not reach the thresholds of major depression.

- Some patients have episodes of mild depression.
- Some patients have a very brief episode of depression. The choice of 2 weeks to define major depression is arbitrary.
- Some depressions are severe but intermittent, each episode lasting under 2 weeks – the so-called recurrent brief depression.

2. Lifelong, mild fluctuating depression, or dysthymia, on which major depressive episodes may be superimposed.
3. Mixed subclinical states falling short of these.
4. Bipolar depression or manic depression, where episodes of depression alternate with mania, is rarely seen. It tends to be severe and is likely to be recurrent.

How common is depression?

Major depression

Around 5% of the adult population will have a major depressive episode during a given year,[3] and of these roughly half will come to medical attention.[2] In deprived areas the prevalence of major depression tends to be higher.

Women are affected twice as often as men.[4]

Around 20% of patients consulting their GP with a new complaint have some depressive symptoms.[4] Of these, 5% have major depression, 5% have milder episodes and 10% have some depressive symptoms.[2]

The lifetime risk of major depression is about a third.[2] The commonest ages are for women 35–55, and for men 45–65.

Other depression

A total of 60–70% of people have depressive symptoms which fall short of major depression at some time in their lives.[3]

Each GP with a list of 2500 will have 400 patients depressed but not consulting, 100 depressed and consulting, 10 referred to a psychiatrist, 2 in hospital, 3–4 attempted suicides and 1 suicide every 4 years.[5]

Who is at risk of depression?

A number of risk factors which are associated with a higher chance of depression have been identified by research. Their presence should further alert the GP to the possibility of a depressive illness.

- Social deprivation.[4]
- Early loss of a parent.
- Having lots of dependants.
- Living in poor housing conditions.
- Working full-time – this applies only to women.
- Members of ethnic minority groups.
- A family history of depression.
- Alcohol abuse or a family history of alcohol abuse.

How can you diagnose depression?

Fifty per cent of depression is missed by GPs at the first consultation. A further 10% is picked up at subsequent consultations, and 20% remits during contact with the GP. This means that the average GP misses 40% of depression completely, of which half gets better without intervention, leaving 20% undetected 6 months later.[2] Patients whose depression is recognized and treated have a better outcome than those in whom the diagnosis is missed.[2]

Can the doctor get better at diagnosing depression?

A number of features are associated with doctors who are more likely to make a diagnosis of depression.[6] Consultation techniques can be improved by feedback through the use of video recording.[2]

- Show empathy.
- Be sensitive to emotional cues.
- Use appropriate psychological questions and probes.
- Ask for clarification of patient complaints.
- Make early eye contact with the patient.
- Assume receptive postures.

Which depressed patients are more difficult to diagnose?

A number of patient features predict a missed psychological diagnosis:

1. Presentation of somatic complaints. Around 25% of depressed patients have somatic symptoms, but only 9% have exclusively somatic symptoms.[4]
2. A coexisting physical disorder is presented.
3. Patient beliefs:[6]
   - GPs do not deal with psychiatric problems.
   - GPs have neither the time nor the inclination to help.
   - Somatic problems can't have a psychological cause.
   - The GP does not need to know.
   - The GP will reject or dismiss the problem.

Patients who present physical symptoms which have psychological causes are said to somatize. Only a minority will have exclusively physical symptoms, so in most patients it is possible to concentrate more attention on the psychological symptoms without seeming to ignore the presenting complaints. The diagnosis of depression has to be negotiated with the patient.

What can you do if you suspect depression?

Some patients will make it easy for you and tell you they are depressed right from the outset. In others the possibility of depression will only come to light at the end of a list of other problems, during which the patient may be 'testing you out' to see if he or she dares to get on to the more sensitive issues. Other patients may know too well they are depressed, but do not want a number of physical manifestations being dismissed as 'due to nerves' or 'all in your head' without proper evaluation.

As well as receptive attitudes, the use of standardized questions is known to make a psychological diagnosis more likely.[4] A joint project called Defeat Depression was launched by the Royal College of Psychiatrists and the Royal College of General Practitioners in 1992. It advocated the use of checklists to detect depression more accurately.

The Goldberg scales[7] were developed in Manchester for GP use, and correlate well with cases identified by DSM-III-R.

Score 1 for each question:
1. Have you had low energy?
2. Have you had loss of interest?
3. Have you lost confidence in yourself?
4. Have you felt hopeless?

If the score is 2 or more, then proceed to:

5. Have you had difficulty concentrating?
6. Have you lost weight (due to poor appetite)?
7. Have you been waking early?
8. Have you felt slowed up?
9. Have you tended to feel worse in the mornings?

A total score of 4 or more indicates a 50% chance of a clinically important depression. Using this scoring system in conjunction with an assessment of the presenting problems will give good diagnostic accuracy.

How can you assess the risk of suicide?

Suicide is the most important complication of depressive illness. All depressed patients should be assessed for the risk of them committing suicide. Assessing the risk with confidence can be very difficult. In practice, if you feel any doubts for the safety of the patient, then advice should be sought, usually from a specialist colleague.

Ask

The patient should be asked about suicidal intentions and will usually tell you. Asking does not give the patient the idea. Nearly all depressed patients will have wondered what would happen if they were no longer alive, and are usually quite relieved to discuss these feelings. Suicidal thoughts are common, but if specific plans are being made, tablets collected, etc., then the risk is great and admission to hospital should be considered.

The idea that patients who talk about suicide are unlikely to do it is false.[8] Having someone to share your innermost thoughts with, however, can be beneficial.

Most people who commit suicide have in retrospect a recognizable psychiatric disorder, but not always depression. The seriousness of the disorder does not correlate well with the suicide risk level.

Sociological risk factors

Epidemiological studies have revealed groups in which a completed suicide is more likely:[4]

- Male patients.
- Older people. Historically this has been true, but currently there is a trend for younger males to kill themselves, possibly as a response to problems with acquired immune deficiency syndrome (AIDS).
- Coexisting physical illness, especially if associated with a lot of pain.
- Socially isolated, particularly living alone.

And additionally in women:

- Loss of mother by death or separation before age 12.
- Three or more children under 5.
- Lack of either a close caring relationship or a job.

Psychological risk factors

- Persistent intense feelings of hopelessness or helplessness.
- Previous attempts at self-harm.
- Alcohol abuse, or family history of abuse.
- Impulsive personality.
- Marked sleep disturbance.
- Family history of mental illness or suicide.

Is admission needed?

The genuinely suicidal patient is a danger to him- or herself in the meaning of the Mental Health Act 1983, and so is liable to compulsory admission.

In a well-supported patient who is less actively suicidal, it may be possible to avoid admission. Any medication should only be dispensed in small quantities, or should be entrusted to a carer. Regular and frequent review is needed.

If you are in any doubt about the need for admission, then further advice should be sought without delay from a specialist colleague. Many psychiatric departments operate a crisis service where patients causing concern can be assessed with the minimum of delay.

Many suicides occur in the early hours of the morning when typically the depressive symptoms are at their worst. This should be borne in mind when seeing a depressed patient in an evening surgery. If there is a suicide risk, it may not be at its greatest when you see the patient. It also does not give you much time to get a second opinion before the next danger time.

What is the initial management of a depressed patient?

Ninety-five per cent of depression is treated in general practice. When compared with consultant psychiatric care, the results are just as good, and are achieved at about half the cost.[9]

All forms of treatment work better in the more severely depressed patient. The effectiveness of treatment in degrees of depression which fall short of major depression is not as good. The *DSM-III-R* criteria therefore also define who is likely to benefit from antidepressant treatment.

Show empathy

Most depressives feel guilty and worthless and will be trying very hard to make themselves feel better. Depression is a common illness, but is surrounded by many taboos. The patient's friends and relations will often, with the best of intentions, be telling the patient to 'shake yourself out of it' or 'pull yourself together'. The general effect of this is to make the sense of guilt worse.

Get the first consultation right

A lot of work has to be done during the first consultation. Many depressed patients feel guilty because of their illness, and so will not want to trouble the doctor with what they will see as their problem. The patient will have worked very hard just to come and talk about the symptoms. If rejected, the illness may submerge for ever or else convert into what the patient may feel are more acceptable physical symptoms.

Most patients will present for the first time at ordinary surgery. Although the initial assessment of the depressed patient can be time-consuming, that time must be taken as it may be the last chance you get. If the full time cannot be spent there and then, having secured the safety of the patient and assured him or her that the problem is real and can be helped, it is reasonable to make an early appointment within the next day or so to complete the job.

Tasks for the first consultation are:

• Listen to the symptoms. This will indicate the diagnosis and also forms a basis by which progress can be assessed at later contacts.
• Enquire about specific biological features of depression, or use a depression scoring checklist.
• Let the patient know what you think the diagnosis is, and give him or her time to react to this suggestion.
• Tell the patient that depression is common, and that it can be treated.
• Explain that family and friends may have difficulty understanding how the patient feels at the moment. Thoughts are disordered, so that how the patient perceives reality is temporarily different from the way everybody else sees it.
• Depression is a real illness with demonstrable chemical changes in the brain. There is no 'badge of office' such as a scar or a plaster cast, but the illness is real none the less. Unfortunately, it distorts your ability to think straight, and this makes the symptoms much worse as you feel personally responsible for being ill.

Put together a support strategy

In all cases, whatever other type of treatment is used, it is important to maintain good therapeutic links with the depressed patient. Encouragement can be offered and progress reviewed. Good practice would include the following:

• See other members of the family, or friends.
• Advise on environmental change; holidays, less stressful work, organizing domestic stresses better.
• Recommend self-help groups.
• Be a patient's advocate. Be prepared to support the patient's interests with other people.
• Set an agenda for change. Delineate problem areas. Encourage the involvement of the patient.

- Discuss other problems, even if you can't do much about them. Talking can help.
- Involve other health workers where appropriate. If you have ready access to a community psychiatric nurse or counsellor, then his or her services can prove invaluable. An early assessment is particularly useful.

What follow-up is required?

The depressed patient needs to be followed-up until better and off treatment. This can be done by the GP at home or in surgery, or by the community psychiatric nurse or health visitor if available.

The frequency of contacts depends on the severity of the depression and the response to treatment. Severe depression with possible suicidal risk will need review every 2 or 3 days unless the patient is to be admitted. Without suicidal risk, review at weekly intervals is appropriate.

For lesser degrees of depression, follow-up can be arranged with reference to what you feel the patient requires. It will take 3 or 4 weeks before any tricyclics start to work, and review before this time may end up in an action replay of the first consultation. If the first consultation has been performed properly, there is little value in this. It wastes everybody's time, and may even make the depression worse by dwelling on the symptoms and reinforcing the fact that treatment has not yet helped.

If the side-effects of medication are too severe to tolerate, advise the patient to come in before the appointed time. It is no good seeing a patient after 4 weeks to assess the results of treatment to find that he or she was only taking the tablets for 2 days.

Tasks for follow-up consultations include:

- Is the medication being tolerated? Most patients who are taking tricyclic antidepressants in effective dosages will be subject to anticholinergic side-effects. The dose or type of medication may need adjusting.
- Has there been a change in symptoms? To avoid getting bogged down in new symptoms it is useful to concentrate on the symptoms presented in the first consultation. If improved, this may be used as positive evidence for you and the patient that treatment is beginning to work. The patient may well not feel on top of the world, but progress is being made. Treatment can only restore patients to their normal mental state, which for most people includes times when they feel better and times when they feel worse.

- Have any changes been implemented which would minimize stress and maximize support? This may include attendance at a self-help group or discussion with members of the family and employers about the problem.
- How are the family and friends reacting? It may not have been possible to explain the patient's illness to other family members, and they may not understand the patient's trouble. It is not uncommon for a patient to be told by a well-intentioned but misguided family member to 'throw your tablets down the toilet'. This is unhelpful.

Medication: what are the options?

Drug treatment is most likely to help patients with more severe forms of depression, though drugs can also be useful in milder illness. Drug treatment can reasonably be considered for all degrees of depression. Drugs should, however, only be used in addition to the support strategies described above. There is no justification in merely issuing a prescription and then letting the patient get on with it.

The patient who declines medication or who seems to get lots of side-effects from treatment may be expressing the guilt of the illness. Being firm and positive is often justified.

Tricyclic antidepressants (TCAs)

These are the oldest preparations. Up to 65% of depressed patients will respond fully or partially to TCAs.[10] Different compounds differ in terms of sedation and cost: amitriptyline is the cheapest and dothiepin the commonest. Clomipramine is useful for phobic and obsessional states. All are toxic in overdosage, and may cause arrhythmias.

Anticholinergic side-effects are almost inevitable if the best result is to be secured. It is reasonable to increase the dose to the maximum tolerated over the course of 1 or 2 weeks. The licensed dose is up to 150 mg/day, or 200 mg in exceptional cases. It is common not to use large enough doses: doses under 75 mg/day have not been shown in controlled trials to help depression,[2] though individual patients may respond to smaller doses and relapse if the medication is stopped.

TCAs take 3–6 weeks to start working. Only if a 6-week trial on full dosage has failed should a change in treatment be considered.

Mianserin

Mianserin is no more effective than TCAs, but is less toxic in overdose. The elderly need monthly full blood counts in the early stages of treatment because of the slight risk of blood dyscrasias. The dose is 30–90 mg/day in a single or divided dose. It is moderately sedative. Mianserin costs more than TCAs.

Lofepramine

Lofepramine is less toxic than the TCAs, but it is no more effective and costs more – about 10 times the cost of amitriptyline. The dose is 140–210 mg/day in divided doses. It is mildly sedative.

Monoamine oxidase inhibitors (MAOIs)

MAOIs can be useful where a quick response to treatment is wanted, or other treatments have proved too sedative or ineffective. Phenelzine has the fewest side-effects (stimulation and dependence). Interactions with food may cause a hypertensive crisis, but the danger of this is exaggerated – only 17 cases were reported over a 10-year period when the use of MAOIs was at its peak. Even so, all recipients should have a diet card and be warned about drug interactions.

MAOIs are useful for depression and somatic anxiety. Compared to tricyclics, they work more quickly, are less sedating, and may work where tricyclics don't. Overall there is a 70% response rate to MAOIs.[11]

Lithium

Lithium is particularly useful in bipolar (manic) depression. Adding lithium to tricyclics improves symptoms in 50–60% of resistant cases.[10] Blood monitoring is needed to avoid side-effects such as gastrointestinal disturbance, blurred vision and drowsiness.

There are important toxic interactions between lithium and angiotensin-converting enzyme inhibitors, non-steroidal anti-inflammatory drugs, selective serotonin re-uptake inhibitor (SSRI) antidepressants, methyldopa and loop diuretics.[12]

Selective serotonin re-uptake inhibitors

These are no more effective than other drugs,[13] but have fewer side-effects such as weight gain (they are actually licensed for use in bulimia), anticholinergic effects and cardiac arrhythmias. SSRIs are much safer in overdosage than TCAs.

SSRIs are about 30 times more expensive than amitriptyline. There is a toxic interaction with lithium.

An attempt has been made to market SSRIs as first-line drugs for depression on the basis of safety and side-effect profile. In trials, there have been as many drop-outs as with tricyclic treatment. TCAs are certainly more toxic in overdose, being responsible for 7% of poisoning deaths in the UK.

Using SSRIs routinely as first-line treatment would cost the NHS £100m a year at 1993 prices.[2]

Flupenthixol

Flupenthixol is a phenothiazine derivative. It is not a powerful antidepressant, but it is quick-acting. Small doses are used when compared to its use as a major tranquillizer.

How long should drug treatment go on?

Depression is a relapsing illness, with episodes tending to get closer together. Twelve per cent of cases evolve into a chronic course.[2] Any patient who has had a depressive illness needs supervision for life. This is best done by getting the patient to report any recurrence of symptoms.

Patients may also need drug treatment for life, sometimes for chronic depression and sometimes to stop the next attack. Episodes need treatment for up to a year, or at least until 4–6 months after resolution of the symptoms.[2]

Relapse rates are 50% at 2–8 months on placebo, and 20% on continued tricyclics,[2] reducing to 10% if brief psychotherapy and family education are added.

In recurrent depression, 80% of patients will have another episode within 2 years; maintenance treatment cuts this to 20% and low-dose maintenance to 50%. In a patient with a second depressive episode, long-term treatment and follow-up should be considered.

What are the options for non-drug treatment?

Cognitive therapy

Cognitive therapy was developed by Beck in the USA. The idea is to try and combat the negative thoughts of depression. The treatment needs a trained therapist and is time-consuming – a usual course lasts 15 hours. It is no more effective than drugs, and there is no added effect when used with drugs. It is, however, useful where drugs are contraindicated or not accepted. There is a 20–38% drop-out rate.[14]

Interpersonal therapy

This is designed to improve or compensate for lack of social contacts and support. It is no more effective than drugs,[14] but is effective alone, especially in the severely depressed.

Electroconvulsive therapy (ECT)

ECT has had a very bad press of late because it is a passive treatment, causes memory loss and is occasionally used compulsorily. However, it works well and quickly, especially in the elderly. An improvement is seen in up to half of cases where tricyclics have failed.

What do the patients think of treatment?

A total of 73% of the general public believe that depression is a medical condition, 46% think antidepressants work, and 78% think they are addictive. Eighty-five per cent think counselling is an effective remedy. Seventy per cent think that GPs are inadequately trained to deal with depressive illness.[15]

About 20–30% of patients will default from drug treatment, and many more will not take it as prescribed.[3,9] However, drop-out rates from non-drug treatments are equally high. In terms of initial patient acceptability, supportive counselling has most appeal. Cognitive therapy can prove difficult for the timid and inarticulate. The idea of drug treatment holds least appeal for the depressed patient; however, it is much more readily available than the alternatives.

Special cases

Children

Ten per cent of 10-year-olds have 'misery', and 1.4% of 10-year-olds and 4% of 14-year-olds are depressed. First-line treatment is psychological, including family therapy. Drugs may work. Suicide risk is low.[16]

The elderly

Three per cent are affected. Symptoms are often masked by physical problems and low expectations. Tricyclics are as effective for both acute attack and preventing relapse. ECT may also be helpful. Remember the possibility of depression when dealing with an elderly patient.[17]

Which patients will benefit from referral?

A GP referral to a psychiatrist costs an average of about £90 for a first visit, and £40 a visit thereafter (1992 prices).[3]
    A domiciliary visit from a psychiatrist costs £100.
    A counsellor employed in general practice costs £15–35 per hour.
    Psychotherapy costs £170 for a first visit, and £80 a visit after.
    Referral should be considered when:[2]

- The diagnosis is in doubt. Is there an underlying organic cause?
- There is significant suicidal risk.
- The patient is unsafe to be left at home because of the severity of the symptoms, because of psychosis, or because there is insufficient family support.
- First-line treatment fails.
- Children.
- Access to additional treatment is needed.
- Bipolar disorder.
- Other psychiatric morbidity coexists, e.g. alcohol dependence or eating disorder.

Can depression be prevented?

The government, through its *Health of the Nation* initiative,[18] has highlighted mental health as one of the five areas targeted for improvement. In particular it has suggested goals of:
- Improving the health and social functioning of mentally ill people.
- Reducing the overall suicide rate by at least 15% by the year 2000 (from 11.1 per 100 000 in 1990 to no more than 9.4 per 100 000).
- Reducing the suicide rate of severely mentally ill people by at least 33% by the year 2000 (from 15% in 1990 to 10%).

The recognition of depressive illness is an important part of this strategy, and clearly an area where the GP is in the best position to respond. If depression is recognized and treated early, then it is briefer and less severe. It seems likely, however, that the primary prevention of depression depends more on social circumstances than on medical care. This is a task for the policy-makers.

Can suicide be prevented?

The assessment of the risk of self-harm is a normal part of the management of the depressed patient. A 1994 review of possible strategies for the prevention of suicide[8] concluded that evidence of effectiveness is lacking, but after further evaluation the following might be considered:

- Targeting patients recently discharged from psychiatric hospital.
- Education of GPs on the recognition and treatment of depression and highlighting the drugs most often taken in fatal overdosage.
- Guidelines on the appropriate management and treatment of depression.
- Schemes to limit the size of individual prescriptions and dose per tablet of high-risk drugs.
- Limitation of the quantity and packaging of aspirin and paracetamol.
- Reinforcement of media guidelines on the reporting and showing of fictionalized suicide.
- Audit of suicide and parasuicide.
- Modification of car exhaust design.

Currently around 25% of people who commit suicide contact a primary care professional (usually the GP) in the week before death, and 40% in the month before.[8] This is a reduction from about 65% 20 years ago and reflects the current trend for younger males to kill themselves deliberately.

The GP is thus in a pivotal position in the recognition of depression, its treatment and in the assessment of suicidal risk. Not all the interventions which might prevent suicide are in the GP's remit, however. The use of a particular method of suicide depends on availability. If a method is widely available, such as the use of coal gas before natural gas was widespread, this itself pushes the suicide rate up. The availability of the means to commit suicide with respect to patient-bought medication and car exhaust fumes will require legislation if it is to be altered.

References

1. American Psychiatric Association. *Diagnostic and Statistical Manual of Mental Disorders*, 3rd edn, revised. Washington, DC: American Psychiatric Association. 1987
2. Paykel ES & Priest RG. Recognition and management of depression in general practice: consensus statement. *Br Med J* 1992; **305**: 1198–202
3. The treatment of depression in primary care. *Effective Health Care* 5 March 1993
4. Wright AF. *Depression: Recognition and Management in General Practice*. London: Royal College of General Practitioners. 1993
5. Martin P. Depression: a GP's perspective. *Update* 1992; **45**: 576–7
6. Boardman J. Detection of psychological problems by general practitioners. *Update* **42**: 1067–73
7. Goldberg D, Bridges K, Duncan-Jones P *et al.* Detecting anxiety and depression in a general practice setting. *Br Med J* 1988; **297**: 897
8. Gunnell D & Frankel S. Prevention of suicide: aspirations and evidence. *Br Med J* 1994; **308**: 1227–33
9. Scott AIF & Freeman CPL. Edinburgh primary care depression study. *Br Med J* 1992; **304**: 883–7
10. Cowen PJ. Depression resistant to tricyclic antidepressants. *Br Med J* 1988; **297**: 435
11. Bass C & Kerwin R. Rediscovering monoamine oxidase inhibitors. *Br Med J* 1989; **298**: 345
12. *British National Formulary* 27. London: British Medical Association Royal Pharmaceutical Society of Great Britain. 1994
13. Song F, Freemantle N, Sheldon TA *et al.* Selective serotonin reuptake inhibitors: meta-analysis of efficacy and acceptability. *Br Med J* 1993; **306**: 683–7
14. Gelder MG. Psychological treatments for depressive disorders. *Br Med J* 1990; **300**: 1087
15. Sims A. The scar that is more than skin deep: the stigma of depression. *Br J Gen Pract* 1993; **43**: 30–1
16. Black D. Depression in children. *Br Med J* 1987; **294**: 462–3
17. Treating depression in the elderly. *Drug Ther Bull* 1989; pp 268–72
18. Secretary of State for Health. *Health of the Nation: A Strategy for Health in England*. London: HMSO. 1992

For a condensed review, see Khot, A. and Polmear, A. *Practical General Practice*, 1992; 2nd edn. Oxford: Butterworth-Heinemann. pp 268–72.

6

Dizzy spells and vertigo

Aims

The trainee should:

- Be aware of the differential diagnosis of dizziness.
- Be able to take an adequate history.
- Have proper regard to time constraints and time management.
- Have knowledge of the available therapeutic options.

Preamble

Balance is the sense of continuity which a person has with his or her environment. Correct balance requires:[1]

- Accurate sensory information from the eyes, proprioceptive receptors (in the joints) and the vestibular labyrinth.
- Accurate coordination of the sensory input by the brain.
- Functioning motor output from the central nervous system to a normal musculoskeletal system.

If one or more of these is not working properly, then a sense of imbalance will result.

When consulting with a patient, it is important to establish what precisely he or she means by the term dizziness:

- *Vertigo* is when patients have a sensation of movement either of themselves or of their surroundings. In its mildest form it may present as a rocking sensation.
- *Syncope* or *Presyncope* is the sensation of an impending faint – a light-headed feeling which may lead to a full-blown syncopal episode.

Some patients will describe a sense of loss of balance or disequilibrium, or other feelings which they may call dizziness but which are neither syncopal nor vertiginous. In practical terms, the most important distinctions to establish are between vertigo, impending faints and everything else. If there has been a witness to a dizzy spell then there may be a further description of the effects of the episode, the presence of pallor and sweating, etc. If consciousness has been lost, a witness is particularly useful.

Dizzy spells in general practice

On average each GP will see 5 or 6 new cases of dizziness per year, as well as many more cases of ongoing dizziness. Of the new cases where a physical diagnosis is made:[2]

- 80% are due to vestibular neuronitis or benign positional vertigo.
- 15% are due to Ménière's disease or vertebrobasilar insufficiency.
- 3% are due to transient ischaemic attack.
- 1% are due to ear infections.
- 1% are due to other causes, including multiple sclerosis.

In addition to these physical causes, other patients will present with dizziness brought on by psychological causes such as anxiety and functional disorders. These constitute the second commonest reason for patients to present with dizziness.

All cases of dizziness cause distress, often to a considerable and disabling extent. Confidence will be lost, and work or favoured hobbies cannot be pursued. Most causes of dizziness are self-limiting and not serious, but very occasionally there may be a more serious cause.

The GP's aim when approached by a patient with dizzy spells must be to make as confident a diagnosis as possible. This will make sure that a serious diagnosis has not been missed, and that any treatment is more likely to work. Most patients with dizziness will fear a brain tumour. The ability to establish a clear alternative diagnosis will help with your attempts to reassure the patient.

At first presentation it is not only necessary to take a sufficient history, but also important that a minimum examination is performed. All this usually means that the consultation will take longer than average. You may as well settle in for the duration as time spent at the first presentation will pay dividends later on.

Common causes of dizziness

Most of the causes of dizziness seen in general practice are managed entirely within general practice. Textbooks written by consultants are often misleading, as in hospital practice they will be seeing a highly selected population with a quite different distribution of pathologies.

Knowledge of a few commonly occurring conditions will cover the vast majority of the cases seen. A symptom pattern which deviates from these common diagnoses will alert the careful practitioner to the occasional more serious diagnosis.

Vestibular neuronitis

This is one of the commonest causes of true vertigo seen in general practice. Around 2 cases per 1000 population per year may be expected. The average age of onset is 40 years (range 20–60), though there is an identical condition which affects children (benign paroxysmal vertigo of childhood). The condition is probably due to an isolated temporary lesion of the vestibular nerve and its connections.

Clinical features
Clinical features are:

• Vertigo, usually severe.
• Absence of cochlear symptoms – deafness and tinnitus.
• Absence of neurological symptoms.

The vertigo comes on quite suddenly and without warning. It is continuous, though it may be of variable severity. Head movements may bring about a worsening of symptoms. Ninety per cent of patients have nausea, and 55% have vomiting. Seventy per cent of patients show nystagmus when tested.[3]

The vertigo lasts for an average of 6 weeks, but symptoms lasting for up to 9 weeks are not unknown. In 43% of cases, attacks are recurrent over months or years.[3] Recurrence is more likely in the younger patients and in those with a more severe initial attack. Each successive recurrence is milder than the one before.

Vestibular neuronitis is preceded by an infectious illness in 45% of cases,[3] and sinusitis in particular may precede an attack. It is also not uncommon for attacks to occur in little epidemics, and in family contacts of sufferers. However, there is no evidence of a direct viral cause for the disorder, though some authorities have postulated an unidentified neurotoxin produced by infection. Most patients are told that their symptoms are due to a viral infection and, though this is not strictly true, it none the less emphasizes the self-limiting nature of the illness.

Treatment

Treatment is partly by vestibular sedation, and partly by the brain compensating for the distorted input it is getting from the vestibular nerve.

- *Explanation and reassurance* are an important part of management. This is a frightening condition, and many patients fear a more severe cause for their symptoms. Specific anxieties should be explored and dealt with.
- *Medication* is used in most cases. Prochlorperazine in a dose of 5 mg three times a day is most useful. If vomiting is prominent, it can also be given by injection or suppository. Other phenothiazine derivatives can be used as alternatives.

  All the phenothiazines and their derivatives can cause acute dystonic reactions, and a Parkinson's-like syndrome on chronic use, which usually but not always abates when treatment is stopped. The elderly are at particular risk, and so these medications should be used with particular caution.

- *Compensation.* In time the brain adjusts to the distorted information it is getting from the labyrinth. This process can be accelerated by doing exercises which tend to bring on the vertigo. At first, eye, head and shoulder movements can be used. When the patient is ambulant, further exercises encouraging bending, upper body movements and games involving rotating and catching are advised. Standing and walking with the eyes closed also stress labyrinthine function. The Cawthorne–Cooksey exercises[4] are a structured form of suitable exercises and can be taught by the physiotherapist in the team.

Benign positional vertigo (BPV)

This condition affects an older age group, being commonest from the fifth decade onwards.[5] Around 25% of cases of dizziness presenting in general practice will have this diagnosis.

Clinical features
Clinical features are:

- Brief severe episodes of vertigo lasting less than a minute.
- The vertigo is provoked by sudden changes of head position, for example looking up, turning the head, or sitting up in bed.
- The reaction decays so that repeating the movement causes less vertigo.

Test
The test of choice[1] can be performed in general practice, but is usually unnecessary since the diagnosis can be obtained from a careful history:

- Sit the patient on a couch with the head turned to face you.
- With the head still turned, lower the patient so that his or her head is over the top edge of the couch and 30% below the horizontal.

Nystagmus provoked by this test is always an abnormal finding. In BPV:

1. Nystagmus is rotatory, beating towards (i.e. fast phase) the downward ear. The direction does not alter during observation.
2. A latent period of several seconds precedes onset.
3. Nystagmus abates after a maximum of 50 seconds (so-called adaptation).
4. Violent vertigo accompanies the nystagmus.
5. On repeating the test, the response diminishes.

The symptoms persist for an average of 6 months, then resolve.[5] Recurrence is not uncommon. The underlying cause is the displacement of calcium crystals (otoliths) in the inner ear. Head movement makes the crystals move about, inducing the symptoms.

Treatment
Treatment begins by explaining the benign nature of the condition. The Cawthorne–Cooksey exercises may be used as a way of getting the brain to compensate. A refinement of this is called habituation, where the patient actively seeks out the head positions which provoke the symptoms. Repeatedly inducing the dizziness accelerates compensation, and 90% success has been alleged.[5]

Medication is commonly prescribed, with prochlorperazine leading the field. With regard to the age group concerned, fears over dystonia should temper pharmacological zeal.

Ménière's disease

This is a disorder of endolymph control causing dilatation of the endolymphatic spaces in the membranous labyrinth. About 1 in 1000 people contract the disease, the commonest ages of onset being 30–60.[1] It usually affects only one ear, but in 20–30% both ears are affected, with correspondingly more severe symptoms and consequences.

Because the underlying problem is in the labyrinth, both the balance and hearing modalities are affected.

Clinical features
Clinical features are:

- Sudden attacks of severe vertigo, often with prostration and vomiting.
- Hearing impairment (sensorineural deafness) and tinnitus in the affected ear.

Attacks last for a minimum of 10 minutes and a maximum of 12 hours.[1] After the attack the tinnitus and deafness may not completely abate, so that after successive attacks the hearing problem is progressively greater.

Attacks often occur in clusters, with interim remissions.[4] The patient may get a warning that the attack is going to start, by a change in the character of the tinnitus, or a sensation of pressure in the ear.

Diagnosis
Diagnosis is made from the history. Apart from the deafness there are no clinical findings between attacks.

Treatment
Treatment is by using vestibular sedatives such as prochlorperazine. In addition, betahistine in a dose of 8–16 mg thrice daily is a vasodilator which reduces endolymph pressure, and thus has a specific role in Ménière's disease.

Severe attacks with vomiting may require injections or suppositories, and in some cases fluid replacement and bedrest are needed.

If attacks cannot be controlled, then the endolymph can be surgically decompressed, a procedure which preserves hearing and relieves vertigo in 80% of cases.[4] If there is no useful hearing left, labyrinthectomy can be performed, and this always stops subsequent vertigo.

Basilar artery migraine

Rarely, migraine affects the basilar artery territory. If it does, then the characteristic migraine headache is preceded by a sudden onset of vertigo. There is often a positive family history. In addition, in 70% of cases the headache is accompanied by giddiness,[6] which in a third of cases is vertiginous.

Once a diagnosis has been made, treatment is as for any other type of migraine. Prophylaxis may be required at an earlier stage because of the dangers of a sudden onset of disabling vertigo when driving or operating machinery.

The development of neurological symptoms associated with migraine contraindicates further use of the combined oral contraceptive pill.

Vertebrobasilar insufficiency (VBI)

This condition is found in an older age group, and there is often a history of other cardiac or vascular disorders. The dizziness produced may or may not be vertigo.

Twenty per cent of sufferers have only dizzy spells,[6] but in the rest there are other neurological symptoms which occur at the same time, such as diplopia, dysarthria and sensory impairment.

Symptoms are brought on by extremes of head movement, often when performing day-to-day tasks.

Treatment is by treating any underlying cause such as hypertension. Failing this, low-dose aspirin can be helpful, as can balancing exercises.

The frail elderly

In the old and frail, falls are common and are an important indicator of impending mortality. The cause of the fall may be described as dizziness but it will not readily fall into one of the categories described above. Descriptions of 'legs going weak', or 'I felt dizzy and I went down' are characteristic.

There is usually a history of more than one degenerative pathology in a patient with poor levels of confidence.[7] Examination will show defects in two or more parts of the balance control system, for instance poor vision, impaired proprioception from arthritis joints and cervical spondylosis. In some cases an additional problem such as a chest infection or mild heart failure can tip the balance and produce falls.

In the context of the frailty, it may be difficult for you and the family to manage the situation at home. An admission for rehabilitation is often needed.

Other reasons for dizziness

The six diagnoses above will cover most of the patients who present with dizziness to the GP. However, there are a number of other possible causes of which it is as well to be aware.

Cardiovascular causes

1. Postural hypotension. A fall in blood pressure of more than 25/15 mmHg on standing confirms the diagnosis. May be drug-induced.
2. Transient ischaemic attack or stroke. Invariably other neurological symptoms are also present.
3. Arrhythmias, Stokes–Adams attacks.
4. Syncope or vasovagal attacks. Pallor and bradycardia accompany a faint feeling. An external stimulus can usually be identified as the cause. A younger age group is affected, the commonest age being during adolescence. Cough and micturition may cause attacks.

Neurological causes

1. Seizures. Grand or petit mal, temporal lobe epilepsy with *déjà vu* and automatism.
2. Brain tumours may present as dizziness, and this will certainly be in the mind of the sufferer. There are invariably other symptoms as well as the dizziness. A cerebellopontine angle tumour – in particular an acoustic neuroma – may be the cause of the vertigo. A brain tumour is not a diagnosis to be missed.
3. Multiple sclerosis will rarely present as dizziness. However, for the small numbers of patients who present under the age of 40, it is rather commoner. Other neurological symptoms are usually present as well.
4. Peripheral neuropathy, which has various causes, can lead to less positional sense in the legs with an attendant feeling of unsteadiness.

Vestibular causes

1. Ear wax may cause dizziness.[8]
2. Seasickness, travel or motion sickness.
3. Acute or chronic middle ear disease.
4. Viral labyrinthitis. A number of viruses may cause this, including mumps, measles, varicella and influenza. There is

an acute onset of hearing loss, vertigo, or both. The condition resolves over a few weeks.

Metabolic
1. Hypoglycaemia.
2. Renal failure.
3. Heart failure.
4. Toxic confusional states; meningitis; pyrexia.

Drugs and alcohol
A number of drugs may cause dizziness through postural hypotension, confusion or direct damage to the labyrinth. Examples include:

• Hypotensives.
• Sedatives.
• Cimetidine, levodopa.
• Analgesics.
• Anticholinergics.
• Eighth nerve damage; frusemide, gentamicin.

Acute alcohol intoxication can present as dizziness and imbalance.

Chronic alcohol abuse may cause imbalance, peripheral neuropathies and eventually Wernicke's encephalopathy.

Psychiatric
1. Vertigo and dizziness are the second commonest neurological symptoms in psychiatric patients, only headache being commoner.[6] Patient will describe a sensation of 'swimmy head' or 'fear of falling', and there is often a feeling of anxiety or fright at the same time. Depressed patients may also present as being dizzy and unable to connect properly with the outside world.
2. Phobic postural vertigo is estimated to be the third commonest cause of vertigo (after vestibular neuronitis and BPV).[6] It affects men aged 30–50 and women aged 20–40 in equal numbers. There is an associated gait disturbance and fear of dying. Triggers such as bridges, tunnels and stairs may be identified as causing the sensations. Early recognition is important to prevent the establishment of an invalid role.
3. Astasia-abasia is a rare psychiatric disorder producing an often quite bizarre gait.

Balance problems
1. Bruns ataxia, a short-stepping broad-based gait with flat feet,

caused by cerebral degenerative conditions, in particular Alzheimer's disease.
2. Parkinson's disease.
3. Cervical spondylosis may cause dizziness, irrespective of any vascular encroachment.

What can the GP do?

When presented with a patient with dizzy spells, it is as well to have a system for establishing the likely diagnosis. Most cases will fall into the group which are eminently managable in general practice. If the history or findings deviate from the normal, however, there are a number of possibly serious reasons for this, and these cases need urgent assessment.

In general the older patients are more likely to have a serious underlying cause for their dizziness. This group is also most vulnerable to the effects of dizziness.

Taking a history

Finding out exactly what has happened will usually point to a diagnosis without the need for much further investigation.

What type of dizziness is it?
True vertigo with a sensation of movement of either the patient or surroundings suggests a disorder either of the labyrinth or of its central connections. The report of a light-headed sensation points to another group of possibilities.

The *duration* of the dizziness is also important. In vestibular neuronitis the vertigo comes on suddenly and persists over several weeks, though it may fluctuate in intensity and in general improve with time. In BPV the dizziness lasts a few seconds or a minute, and then abates. In Ménière's disease, the vertigo lasts a maximum of 12 hours.

The *frequency* of the dizzy spells should be established. Vestibular neuronitis is usually a single, though prolonged, episode, though sometimes there may be recurrences. BPV is recurrent over several months before it remits. Attacks of Ménière's disease occur in crops, but the disease process usually extends over years.

Are there any other symptoms?
Any cause of severe vertigo may lead to nausea and vomiting.

The presence of deafness or tinnitus suggests that the labyrinth is involved in the disorder.

Episodic headaches will point to migraine, but a more persisting headache, especially if other neurological symptoms are present, may indicate a space-occupying cerebral lesion.

Intermittent claudication or angina are signs of generalized vascular problems, so that any dizziness may well be of circulatory origin such as transient ischaemic attack or VBI.

Does anything make the dizziness better or worse?
Dizziness brought on by head movements will suggest BPV or VBI. Dizziness when standing up may be due to postural hypotension, and on prolonged standing may be a vasovagal attack.

Are you taking any pills or medicines?
These may be prescribed or otherwise, therapeutic or otherwise. The elderly patient is at particular risk of dizziness due to drug side-effects or interactions. An assessment of alcohol consumption is helpful.

Do you feel anxious or depressed?
Psychological pathology may be the cause of or the result of dizziness.

What do you think may be wrong?
Establishing the patient's agenda is a useful way of making sure that specific fears and concerns have been dealt with. The common fears in patients with dizziness are of brain tumour, multiple sclerosis, hypertension or imminent stroke.

What are the effects of the dizziness?
Sedentary patients may not find their dizziness too troublesome. On the other hand, a lorry driver who has disabling attacks of dizziness without warning is not safe to do his job and secure his livelihood. A favourite hobby may be interfered with, or a household chore rendered impossible.

The examination

1. The *ears* should be examined for evidence of acute or chronic infection, or impacted wax or damage to the drum. If there are symptoms of hearing loss the Rinne test will establish whether it is conductive or sensorineural.
2. A check of the *blood pressure* will not usually be helpful, but

patients will not feel they have been properly examined unless it is measured. Where postural hypotension is suspected, pressure should be measured sitting and standing.

3. A *cardiovascular assessment* may reveal an arrhythmia, abnormal heart sounds, a carotid bruit or anaemia.
4. *Neck movements* should be checked. Dizziness may be provoked, especially at extremes of the range.
5. Where vertigo is present, the patient should be tested for *nystagmus* by direct observation and after postural manoeuvres. The nystagmus of benign conditions is always horizontal and does not alter in direction. Any nystagmus which is not like this is a sign of possible serious pathology.
6. *Balance* can be checked by watching the gait and by having the patient walk with the eyes open and then closed. Romberg's sign is positive when the patient is unable to balance with the eyes closed, and this may point to a cerebellar lesion.
7. *Other examinations* may be suggested by the history.

Investigations

Investigations are not often required. A haemoglobin assay may show evidence of anaemia, and macrocytosis will suggest vitamin B_{12} deficiency. An erythrocyte sedimentation rate assessment may suggest that a significant disease process is occurring. Urea and electrolyte estimation will measure renal function. Urine or blood tests for glucose may detect occult diabetes.

If there is concern about a cause for the dizziness which cannot be dealt with in general practice, further investigation is required. A transient arrhythmia may only be detected on a 24-hour electrocardiogram. Hospital referral will be needed for more specialized investigations or if a serious diagnosis is suspected.

What advice can you give the patient?

Self-care

Accidents can be avoided by removing hazards such as frayed carpets. Footwear with side support (not slippers) will be helpful. Old solid furniture may provide adequate places which can be held for support when walking round the house, but newer light-weight furniture is much less reliable in this respect. Floors should be clear of anything which may be tripped over.

Walking aids in the form of a stick or a Zimmer frame may give confidence. In smaller houses the larger aids may get in the way and it is not unusual to attend on a visit and find a brand new, unused Zimmer parked permanently in a passageway and doing no good. Hand rails on stairs can be of particular use, especially as the stairs in older houses tend to be steep. The local authority can sometimes be persuaded to supply these. Bathing is another hazardous time which can be negotiated more confidently with the use of bath aids. Other aids and adaptations may be advised and supplied through the community occupational therapist.

Activities involving neck extension or quick turns of the head are more likely to bring on many forms of dizziness. Inducing the dizziness to help the brain compensate can be very useful, but there are times such as crossing the road, standing on a chair to get something out of a cupboard, or hanging out the washing when a dizzy spell can be particularly hazardous.

Improved mobility and flexibility will not only improve proprioception, but also make it more likely that a dizzy spell can be compensated for without injury. Balance and general fitness exercises may well be helpful, with additional advice from the physiotherapist.

The presence of a carer or other support can make the difference between independence and not coping.

If a dizzy spell does occur, it is important that the patient knows what to do. Sitting or lying in a place of safety will allow time to elapse while the episode abates. A gentle controlled fall is often safer than grabbing at the nearest piece of furniture so that it falls on top of the patient. Once on the floor, rolling over on to the side and then the front is the best way of preparing to stand, but this need not be attempted until the dizziness has abated. In severe cases a radio alarm which the patient carries round the neck or on the wrist can be most useful and reassuring.

Other help

Practical help and advice for the patient who suffers from dizzy spells may be provided by the home help service, occupational therapist, physiotherapist or chiropodist.

References

1. Ludman H. *ABC of Ear, Nose and Throat*, 2nd edn. London: British Medical Association. 1988; pp. 24–6

2. Fry J. (ed) *Beecham Manual for Family Practice*, 3rd edn. Lancaster: MTP Press. 1985; p. 167
3. Cooper CW. Vestibular neuronitis: a review of a common cause of vertigo in general practice. *Br J Gen Pract* 1993; **43**: 164–7
4. Ludman H. Investigation and treatment of vertigo. *The Practitioner* 1994; **238**: 126–8
5. Denholm SW. Benign paroxysmal positional vertigo. *Br Med J* 1993; **307**: 1507–8
6. Fowler TJ. Assessment and management of vertigo and dizziness. *Update* 1991; **43**: 337–49
7. Overstall PW. A protocol for the diagnosis of balance problems. *Care of the Elderly* 1992; **4**: 174–5
8. Booton P. Diagnosing dizziness. *Update* 1992; **45**: 270–5

Cholesterol and the general practitioner

Aims

The trainee should:

- Know who should have their cholesterol level measured.
- Be able to counsel the patient who requests a cholesterol test.
- Be able to detail a strategy of care for the patient with a raised cholesterol.

Statistics – what is all the fuss about?

Heart attacks kill 180 000 people each year in the UK. Coronary heart disease (CHD) is by far the commonest cause of premature death, being responsible for 36% of all male deaths and 28% of all female deaths.[1]

Cholesterol levels have a linear relationship with CHD risk both within and between populations.[2] It is generally accepted that a 1% lowering of cholesterol will bring about a 2% reduction in the heart attack rate.[3,4]

In the UK only 25% of the population have a serum cholesterol level of under 5.2 mmol/l. Forty per cent have levels between 5.2 and 6.4 mmol/l, 25% have levels between 6.5 and 7.8 mmol/l, and 10% have levels of 7.8 mmol/l or more.[5] People with the highest cholesterol levels run the highest risk of having a heart attack, but there are many more people in the moderate risk group, so that more heart attacks occur in this group.

A number of ways are known of reducing cholesterol levels. Some are concerned with trying to get patients to modify their eating and exercise habits, which is a generally time-consuming and thankless task. Other methods involve the consumption of drugs, and the production of these drugs is a major growth area for the pharmaceutical industry. The prevention of heart attacks is thus medically important and potentially lucrative, securing the continued interest of a large number of people.

The *Health of the Nation*[16] identified CHD as a key area for intervention. Two targets were suggested:

- To reduce the death rate for CHD in people under 65 by at least 40% by the year 2000 (from 58 per 100 000 in 1990 to no more than 34 per 100 000).
- To reduce the death rate for CHD in people aged 65–74 by at least 30% by the year 2000 (from 899 per 100 000 in 1990 to no more than 629 per 100 000).

How to measure cholesterol

1. What to measure

Cholesterol is deposited to form atheromatous plaques. Low-density lipoprotein (LDL) is the major transporter of cholesterol in the blood and largely accounts for the close relationship of cholesterol levels to CHD.[2] Conversely, high-density lipoprotein (HDL) is inversely related to CHD risk. Triglyceride levels are elevated in a number of lipid disorders but, though they may cause pancreatitis, their role in CHD is not clear.

A full lipid assessment should properly measure all these elements. However, a random serum cholesterol level is much easier to obtain as the patient has to be fasted for at least 12 hours before a full profile can be measured. Also most of the major trials have used random cholesterol estimations, so it is the investigation of choice if you want to be able to apply research data to the clinical situation.

2. How to take the sample

It is necessary to take blood samples for cholesterol measurement in a standardized way. A number of things are known to alter a cholesterol assay.[7]

- Posture may alter the reading by up to 10%.
- Occluding the vein for more than 5 minutes can elevate the level by up to 15%.
- Blood taken in the evening can give readings up to 15% higher.
- Readings in winter are around 5% higher than in summer.
- Strenuous exercise in the 2–3 hours before the sample is obtained may also alter the result.

- Blood should be dispatched promptly to the laboratory or the readings will be altered.

Laboratories tend to try and achieve a reading accuracy of plus or minus 5%. Desktop machines are seldom accurate to more than plus or minus 15%, tending to underestimate the true level.

A single cholesterol reading is not very useful. Repeated estimations will regress to the norm, so that high readings will generally come down, and low readings will go up when repeated.

The British Hyperlipidaemia Society[2] has made the following recommendations:

a. Measurements are best performed in hospital chemical pathology departments.
b. Blood should be taken with minimum venous occlusion.
c. Subjects should have been sitting for 10 minutes before the test.

Who should have a cholesterol test?

The whole point of medical interest in cholesterol is to try and reduce the chance of an individual having a heart attack. The risk of having a heart attack is known to be increased by the following factors:[7]

Alterable

- Raised total serum cholesterol level.
- Smoking, especially of cigarettes.
- Hypertension.
- Diabetes mellitus.
- Being overweight.
- Taking insufficient physical exercise.

Unalterable

- Getting older.
- Being male.
- Having a personal history of CHD.
- Having a family history of CHD.

These factors are not just additive, they are synergistic. Looking only at cholesterol levels is a small part of the full picture. Altering a person's cholesterol level if the overall CHD risk is low confers no benefits, and may even cause damage.[8]

In addition, 0.2% of the population have familial hypercholesterolaemia, and another 0.5% have other familial hyperlipidaemias. These people are at particular risk of CHD independently of other risk factors, and also benefit from lipid-lowering treatment.

Therefore the patients who need a cholesterol test are those whose overall CHD risk is high, and those who might have a familial hyperlipidaemia.

Assessing CHD risk

A number of ways of doing this have been suggested. This method is derived from the deliberations of a working party which was establishing a local policy for Sheffield.[9]

In patients who are male and aged 40–60, or female aged 50–60, the following groups should be offered a cholesterol assay:

• Patients who have hypertension.
• Patients who have diabetes.
• Patients with known CHD, or who have chest pain suggesting angina. This symptom should be specifically enquired about as the incidence is probably much greater than is known from medical records.

The assessment of cholesterol levels in the overweight, the underactive and cigarette smokers is controversial. Though they all increase CHD risk, it can also be argued that doing anything about the cholesterol is irrelevant if the other alterable risk factors are not dealt with first.

Assessing the risk of familial hyperlipidaemia

Patients of any age should be tested if they fall into any of the following groups:

• Family history of familial hyperlipidaemia.
• First-degree relative with hyperlipidaemia, xanthelasmata or xanthomata.
• Corneal arcus under the age of 60.
• Family history of CHD under the age of 50.
• Premature vascular disease.

This strategy will detect 30% of those people with a cholesterol level of over 8 mmol/l.

What to do with a cholesterol result

This rather depends on whom you believe. There is now a wealth of data confirming that people with the lowest cholesterol levels run the least risk of having a heart attack. The data also confirm that those at highest risk have most to gain by having their cholesterol levels artificially altered.

Cholesterol under 5.2 mmol/l

This group is at very low risk, whatever their other habits. Remember, however, that any subsequent readings may well be higher because of regression to the mean. General lifestyle advice about smoking, diet and exercise is still desirable.

Cholesterol 5.2–6.4 mmol/l

In the absence of confirmed CHD, this group has little to gain from cholesterol alteration. None the less, lifestyle advice is appropriate. If there is coexisting CHD, then treatment should be considered.

Cholesterol 6.5–7.8 mmol/l

Patients in this group with CHD or multiple risk factors for CHD will benefit from treatment. In the first instance a diet can be recommended. A repeat assay at 3 months will see if the diet has worked, and if not, referral to a dietitian for more specific diet is needed.

Cholesterol 7.9–9.9 mmol/l

This group is at high risk of CHD. These are the sorts of levels found in secondary hypercholesterolaemia (see later), which will necessitate referral. In the absence of an underlying cause, a lipid-lowering diet is indicated. If there is no response at 3 months, referral to a specialized lipid clinic may be helpful, with a view to starting drug treatment.

Cholesterol over 10 mmol/l

These sorts of levels are found in patients with familial hyperlipidaemias. If the level is confirmed, referral to a lipid clinic is needed.

Secondary hyperlipidaemia

A proportion of patients will have a raised cholesterol level because of another underlying disease process. Treatment should initially be directed at the primary disease. Possible culprits are:

- Hormonal, such as pregnancy, diabetes, hypothyroidism.
- Nutritional, such as obesity, anorexia nervosa, alcohol abuse.
- *Hepatic* such as primary biliary cirrhosis, extrahepatic biliary obstruction.
- *Renal* such as nephrotic syndrome, chronic renal failure.
- *Iatrogenic*, such as high-dose thiazides, β-blockers which don't have an α-blocking effect, corticosteroids, retinoids, exogenous sex hormones.

Treatment of raised cholesterol

For some patients it will be concluded, after assessment of their overall CHD risk, that artificially lowering the cholesterol will do some good. Treatment will probably be lifelong, so this is not a decision to be taken lightly.

Smoking

Smoking is by far the most important avoidable risk factor for CHD. Whatever else is done, every effort must be made to encourage the patient to stop smoking. In among the many other cardiovascular risks of cigarette smoking, it also causes serum cholesterol to be slightly raised.

Diet

Diet is the mainstay of treatment for all types of hyperlipidaemia. The aim is to get body weight into the ideal range, and to reduce and alter the amount of fat ingested. Serum cholesterol is made largely from dietary fat, and to a much lesser extent from dietary cholesterol. Also polyunsaturated fats tend to reduce serum cholesterol levels while saturated fats increase them.

The *step one diet* is recommended in the first instance. More rigid diets can be tried if this fails. The step one diet consists of:

- Reducing total fat to less than 30% of calories.
- Changing the ratio of polyunsaturated to saturated fats (the P : S ratio) to 1.0.

- Total dietary cholesterol should be less than 300 mg/day.
- Calories are reduced to achieve a desired weight.

In addition, alcohol intake will need to be within the recommended range (i.e. 21 units a week for a man and 14 units for a woman), or below this if obesity is a problem.

The improvement in cholesterol achievable by the adoption of the step one diet has been reported to be as high as 25%. However, when free-living patients are looked at, the effect is less impressive, with a figure of 2% being more likely.[3] A very rigid diet will lower cholesterol levels substantially, but is very hard to keep to.

Dietary habits are not only a result of patient choice. Availability, palatability (which may well depend on tradition), and cost are also influences. Two authoritative bodies, the British Hyperlipidaemia Society[2] and the King's Fund[10] emphasize the importance of a national food policy if the potential reduction in CHD rate achievable through dietary modification is to be secured.

Exercise

Regular strenuous exercise reduces lipid levels and alters the HDL : LDL ratio in a way which may be helpful.

More modest exercise reduces CHD risk independently of lipid levels. Exercise should be regular, around three times a week and lasting 20 minutes or more. Swimming and brisk walking (4 miles per hour) are ideal as they are aerobic and do not put undue strain on the joints.

Drugs

Medication can be used if other methods of treatment have failed after a trial of at least 6 months.[2]

There was a sixfold increase in the number of prescriptions for lipid-lowering drugs between 1986 and 1992 in the UK[8] and the total annual cost is around £400m. The increase in use in other parts of the world is even greater.

Anion exchange resins
Anion exchange resins have been around for 20 years. They bind bile acids, making the liver produce more and using up cholesterol in the process. Cholesterol levels can be reduced up to 20%, but triglycerides may actually increase.

The two currently available (cholestyramine and colestipol) are in granular form and need to be mixed with water. Gastrointestinal side-effects such as bloating, flatulence and constipation are common, and mean that full compliance with treatment is unlikely. However, in patients who can tolerate them, they are the treatment of choice in isolated raised cholesterol.

Fibric acid derivatives

Fibric acid derivatives are numerous and include bezafibrate, ciprofibrate and gemfibrozil. The parent, clofibrate, causes gallstones so is no longer used. They will reduce triglyceride levels up to 50%, and increase HDL levels up to 20%, but the overall effect on cholesterol is less predictable.

Tolerance is usually good, with mild gastrointestinal symptoms being the only side-effect. Fibrates are drugs of first choice for nearly all lipid disorders.

Nicotinic acid

Nicotinic acid in large doses reduces cholesterol and triglyceride by mechanisms not understood. It is hard to take because of gastrointestinal side-effects and flushing.

Statins

Statins or human menopausal gonadotrophin–coenzyme A (HMG-CoA) reductase inhibitors are the latest, most powerful and by far the most expensive lipid-lowering agents available. They inhibit the liver pathways through which LDL is produced. They are highly effective, with reductions in cholesterol of up to 40% and of triglycerides up to 20% being achievable.

They are palatable and need to be taken only once a day. Side-effects are few; myositis with muscle pain occasionally develops. They are drugs of first choice either alone or with resins in isolated raised cholesterol, and with resins where triglycerides are also elevated.

Once drugs are started, treatment will usually be for life. As well as the costs and monitoring involved, there is also psychological cost because of the creation of a patient. The initiation of drug treatment for hyperlipidaemia is a job for our hospital colleagues either through general medical or specialized lipid clinics.[9]

The great screening debate

In the UK an opportunistic screening programme for raised cholesterol is advised. In the USA, using the same evidence, everyone is advised to have their cholesterol levels checked by the age of 20. Why should different conclusions have been reached? Arguments in favour of mass screening include the following:

- CHD is a very important cause of morbidity and mortality. Even a small reduction in risk will thus save a lot of illness and death.
- The actual incidence of CHD is probably much higher than the known incidence because of so-called silent ischaemia, which is only apparent on electrocardiograph. As pre-existing CHD is a powerful reason for reducing cholesterol, there is a lot of unmet need which will not emerge unless everyone is tested.
- Case-finding for familial hyperlipidaemia is at best 30% effective. Since this group has a lot to gain from treatment, up to 70% will be missed if screening is not routine.

Arguments for opportunistic screening include the following:

- In the UK everyone is registered with a GP. Population coverage of 90% can be achieved in 3 years as this is the proportion of the list which will on average be seen over this period.
- Patients with an overall low CHD risk have little to gain from efforts to reduce their cholesterol. The chance finding of a raised level in someone who is otherwise well creates anxiety and may possibly lead to unnecessary treatment.
- Patients with a normal cholesterol level but other risky habits may be reassured and so not motivated to alter. Even the finding of an abnormal level is unlikely to motivate people to change their habits.[11]
- Major risk factors for CHD are the result of personal habits such as smoking, eating and exercise. These are only partly medical problems. Education and government policy will probably have as much impact as the one-to-one efforts of GPs.

The great treatment debate

Attitudes towards the treatment of raised cholesterol range from the nihilist to the zealot. The evidence available is conflicting and confusing, with many apparent inconsistencies. Some of the dilemmas are:

- CHD risk is linearly related to serum cholesterol level. However, efforts to reduce levels artificially with drug treatments have until recently not been shown to alter the overall death rates in treated groups. Members of treated groups have had more deaths from accidents and suicides than would be expected. The reason for this is not understood but it is postulated that, since fats are important in brain development and function, then alterations in body fat composition may affect either mood or cognitive functions.

- Different groups of patients respond in different ways to drug treatment. Efforts at primary prevention of CHD are less impressive than treatment of those who already have CHD. Men respond better to treatment than women. The older patients respond less well than the younger ones.
- Cholesterol reduction has more effect on non-fatal heart attacks than it does on fatal ones. Death is the only end-point measure which is always free of observer bias, and this gives it considerable authority when used in research.
- Cholesterol reduction by non-drug means seems to have benefits in terms of reduced CHD, but does not appear to carry the possible risks of drug treatments.

Whom can you believe?

A *British Medical Journal* leader in 1994[4] concluded that reducing high cholesterol levels, however it was done, reduces the overall death rate, but this is only apparent after 5 years of treatment. There are no diseases produced by cholesterol-lowering except a small increase in haemorrhagic stroke. Lipid-lowering drugs are generally safe, but this cannot be assumed of newly introduced agents.

References

1. Waine C. The primary prevention of coronary heart disease. *R Coll GP Members' Reference Book* 1989; 183–96
2. Betteridge DJ, Dodson PM, Durrington PN *et al.* for the British Hyperlipidaemia Association. Management of hyperlipidaemia: guidelines of the British Hyperlipidaemia Association. *Postgrad Med J* 1993; **69**: 359–69
3. Ramsay L, Yeo WW and Jackson PR. Dietary reduction of serum cholesterol concentration: time to think again. *Br Med J* 1991; **303**: 953–7
4. Marmot M. The cholesterol papers. *Br Med J* 1994; **308**: 351–2
5. Brown JG. Dietary control of blood cholesterol. *R Coll GP Members' Reference Book* 1989; 319–20
6. Secretary of State for Health. *Health of the Nation: Key Areas Handbook: Coronary Heart Disease and Stroke.* London: Department of Health. 1993

7. McGrath LT. How much faith can you place in a plasma lipid result? *Update* 1992; **45**: 745–56
8. Smith GD, Song F and Sheldon TA. Cholesterol lowering and mortality: the importance of considering initial level of risk. *Br Med J* 1993; **306**: 1367–73
9. Sheffield 2000 Serum Cholesterol Working Party. *Serum Cholesterol Screening Guide*. Sheffield: Sheffield 2000 1991
10. Blood cholesterol measurement in the prevention of coronary heart disease. 6th King's Fund concensus statement. London: Kings Fund Centre 1989
11. Robertson I, Phillips A, Mant D *et al*. Motivational effects of cholesterol measurement in general practice health checks. *Br J Gen Pract* 1992; **42**: 469–72

8

Terminal care at home

Aims

The trainee should:

- Have knowledge of the possible psychological reactions which may occur in an individual or family faced with a terminal diagnosis.
- Have knowledge of the available palliative strategies.
- Be able to structure a care programme, particularly with regard to a team approach.

Statistics

At present, 23% of people in the UK die at home, and 71% in institutions (54% in hospital, 13% in nursing or residential homes and 4% in hospices).[1] At the beginning of the century the vast majority of deaths occurred at home.

According to one study, of those people who are expecting to die, about half would rather die at home, a quarter in hospital and a quarter in a hospice. If home circumstances had allowed, two-thirds of this sample expressed a preference to die at home.[2]

Because people are living longer, more people die when they are elderly. Twenty-five per cent of people live alone,[1] and this group is mainly elderly. Lack of family support is an important reason why people do not die at home.

In 1986 it was estimated that lay carers provided £7.3b worth of informal care.[3] Much of this care is for the terminally ill.

The main carers of the dying person are most commonly wives, husbands and daughters, in that order. As the average age of death rises, so the age of carers goes up. Over 50% of carers are past retiring age.[4]

In their final year of life, 75% of patients spend under 3 months in hospital, 54% under 2 months and 16% under a month. All these figures are falling with time.[1] Even for those who die away from home, much of the terminal care still falls on to community resources.

A GP with an average list size will have about 5 patients each year who die at home. In addition there will be at any one time around 2 patients who are terminally ill and at home.

The psychology of the terminally ill patient

When presented with a fatal diagnosis, people typically undergo a grief reaction very similar to bereavement:

- Initial numbness and denial.
- Anger, bargaining.
- Depression.
- Coming to terms with reality.

Ninety per cent of cancer sufferers want to be told their diagnosis, exact details of their illness and treatment options.[5] It may be upsetting at the time for patient, carers and doctors, but it helps in the adjustment process.

The GP needs to be sensitive to cues for those minority who do not wish to be told the diagnosis. Sometimes it is the carers and other family members who do not want the fatal diagnosis to be disclosed. The wishes of others is not of itself a good reason to withhold information, even though others may give added insight into the character of the patient. A standard strategy is along the lines of: 'I won't tell him the diagnosis, but if he asks I'm not going to tell lies'.

What to say

The majority (up to 80%) of cancer sufferers want to be actively involved in decisions about their treatment. However, only 10% of patients wish to take the major role,[5] presumably so that they are protected from the responsibility for a 'bad decision'. In general the younger, better educated and female are more likely to want to be involved. The desire to participate in management decisions is associated with greater optimism about outcome.[5]

In order to make informed decisions, patients will want to know about various aspects of their disease:

- The nature of any treatment proposed, including the frequency and reversibility of any adverse effects and the expected benefits.

- The duration of treatment and time in hospital.
- Any non-physical effects (depression, loss of libido, family effects).

How to say it

In general, patients with advanced cancer are more likely than their doctors expect, and more likely than healthy people, to opt for major but possibly curative procedures even though there is a risk of severe toxicity and the possible benefits are small.

In choosing treatment options, patients are much influenced by what they believe their doctor wants them to do. Terminally ill patients and their carers consistently rate their quality of life as better than their doctor's estimation. When explaining options, it is important for the doctor not to let his or her own feelings influence how information is presented.

The communication of the fatal diagnosis has to be done carefully. The illness and any medication being taken may cause the patient to be confused. Information has to be specific and concrete. Words used should be understandable.

When breaking bad news, the following may help:[6]

- Make protected time available.
- Deliver information slowly. Pause between pieces of information.
- Be honest without being brutally honest, especially when predicting the effects of treatment. Do not promise what you cannot deliver.
- Try and assess the immediate reaction and answer initial questions at the time. The answers may need to be modified to fit in with how you think the patient is reacting.
- Explore the patient's concerns. This can sometimes be helped by reflecting questions back to the patient. Once identified, additional time either then or at another time should be set aside for further discussion.

In order to make sure that the intended information has been transmitted, explicit categorization may be useful:

1. First say what you are going to say.
2. Then say it.
3. Summarize what you have said.

Written material or a tape recording of the consultation can be taken away by the patient for further reference.

A patient or relative will often request a second opinion to confirm the fatal diagnosis. Such a request should not be regarded as part of a denial process. Occasionally mistakes are made and it is not unreasonable to want further confirmation of such a significant diagnosis. As a patient will often need information from several sources, a second opinion should be encouraged for those who wish it.[5] It does not necessarily mean that the patient has lost faith in your judgement. In practice, it would be rare for a GP to make a terminal diagnosis without confirmation from a hospital colleague.

The psychology of the carers

Carers are usually family members so they will be emotionally affected by the making of a terminal diagnosis. As well as coping with their own reaction, which will usually be very similar to a bereavement reaction, they are also involved in the physical and psychological care of the patient. Putting on a brave face is very common.

Conspiracy of silence

Carers are less willing than doctors to be open about a fatal diagnosis and to discuss death.[6] Carers may affect a jollity and false optimism. The patient usually reacts by thinking that the carers are unable to face up to the imminent death and so they also try and make believe that they are not expecting to die.

At the time when the patient needs the most support from carers, relationships are clouded with lies and deceptions. Getting the patient and carers to talk together openly about their feelings and fears is an important aim for the GP.

The psychology of the professionals

Much of medical training puts so much emphasis on cure rather than care that the death of a patient is regarded as a professional failure. Professionals are also exposed to the same social taboos which surround death. They may have unresolved grief of their own which needs to be dealt with.

These sorts of feelings can cause anxiety for professional carers. Decisions have to be based on what is in the best interests of the patient, and a fatal outcome does not preclude this. It is quite possible to have a good death with all parties satisfied.

Inverse confidentiality

Once a fatal diagnosis has been made, professionals tend to go into 'terminal mode'. The emphasis changes to palliation and there is less concern about drug dependence. Any patient who is not already aware that he or she is dying will almost certainly realize that a change in tactics has occurred.

A respect for the important role which lay carers have plus reservations about being too open with the patient may lead to giving the carers more information than the patient – a sort of inverse confidentiality.

The team

In a terminal care situation new members join the primary health care team and need assimilation. The family are central to the team, and specialist nurses may join the usual nurse/doctor team. Greater efforts at team-building have to be employed, and the sharing of information is particularly important to this.

The Macmillan Service[7] is funded by the National Society for Cancer Relief. Macmillan nurses all have district nurse or health visitor training, and then additional specialist training. They aim to provide a specialist resource, and to develop a relationship with the patient and family. Where available, they can perform a very useful function. Care must be taken, however, to make sure that the existing doctor/district nurse team is not disrupted by the new expert.

Symptom control

Palliative care is defined by the World Health Organization as: 'the active total care of patients whose disease is not responsive to curative treatment'.[8] This emphasizes the active component of the care. Curative treatments need not be suddenly switched to palliative ones: the process is better seen as a gradual shift in emphasis from one to the other.

In 90% of cases where palliative care is needed, the primary diagnosis is of cancer.[8]

Around half of GPs feel that they could benefit from further training in palliative care.[9]

Pain

Eighty per cent of cancer sufferers experience pain.[10] Studies done in the 1960s indicated that the pain of terminal illness was not well-controlled by GPs. Later work suggests that the situation is much improved, with 96% of patients having their pain controlled.[4]

The patient may have more than one type of pain, and may need more than one analgesic intervention.

Regular treatment is required. As-required or PRN regimes are less efficient and also allow the pain to break through. Some have argued that as far as terminal care is concerned, PRN stands for pain relief negligible.

The analgesic ladder

This is the approach recommended by the World Health Organization. It is suggested that pain control should be pursued in a stepwise fashion starting with simple remedies and then progressing to more potent agents if pain is not controlled. At each step, an agent from the appropriate group of drugs can be chosen.

It is no good switching to different preparations in the same group if pain is not controlled; a drug from a stronger group is needed.

1. Mild pain can be relieved by aspirin 600 mg 4-hourly, or paracetamol 1 g every 4–6 hours. These agents may also be added to other regimes on a PRN basis.
2. Moderate pain needs weak opioid preparations such as codeine 30–60 mg 4-hourly, or dihydrocodeine 30 mg 6-hourly. Laxatives should be routinely prescribed.
3. Severe pain needs narcotic analgesia of the strong opiate class. The correct dose is that which works – there is no maximum.

Four-hourly morphine can be used at first to establish the dose required. An ineffective dose should be increased by 50% each time until control is achieved. The total daily dose can then be swapped on to long-acting preparations: for example, 20 mg morphine 4-hourly can be altered to morphine slow-release (such as MST) 60 mg twice a day.

An additional PRN dose of oral morphine can be added in case there is breakthrough pain.

Morphine is the oral preparation of choice. In liquid form it is easily ingested and dosage can be titrated accurately. If taste is a problem, Oramorph has the morphine taste masked. Diamorphine is much more soluble and so is more suitable if injected opiate is needed.

Side-effects such as nausea and sedation often fade over a few days.

Difficult pain

Pain arising from tissue damage is called nociceptive pain. It responds very well to opiates. Other types of pain may, however, be present with or sometimes without nociceptive pain. Bone pain and neurological pain are notoriously resistant to treatment with the agents above.

1. Bone pain will often respond to local radiation or non-steroidal anti-inflammatory preparations.
2. Neurological pain will benefit from tricyclics or antiepileptics.
3. Visceral pain responds poorly to morphine, and indeed may be made worse.[11] Laxatives will ease pain from constipation. Also antispasmodics such as hyoscine may well help.
4. Sympathetic pain is a dull or burning sensation which is hard to localize. The painful area also shows signs of sympathetic overactivity such as erythema and sweating. Antiepileptic drugs can be useful.

It is possible to augment the effect of analgesics with tricyclic antidepressants in standard dosages. A significant number of the terminally ill are depressed anyway, and this symptom may also be helped. It is worth remembering, however, that agents such as tricyclic antidepressants and antiepileptics are not licensed for use in pain control, and so the prescriber takes responsibility for their use.

Route of administration

Medication should be given orally where possible. When this is not possible because of nausea or intestinal obstruction, then other routes have to be found.

Injections are painful, particularly in the emaciated patient. Lack of muscle bulk and circulatory failure may make absorption unreliable.

Many analgesics are available in the form of suppositories, and this is a very efficient route of delivery. However they can be difficult to self-administer and can be ineffective if they induce reflex defecation. Unlike in some countries, the route has never been popular and common in British medical practice.

Syringe drivers can be very useful when the oral route cannot be used. An electrical or sometimes clockwork device slowly delivers a dose of medication over a period of time. Many practices have their own syringe drivers since they are a popular piece of equipment for communities to donate to their local primary care services. Otherwise they can sometimes be borrowed from hospitals or hospices, or even bought by the practice.

A subcutaneous needle is used, and the most suitable drug is diamorphine. The 24-hour dose can be calculated by dividing the amount of morphine taken by mouth by four to get the equivalent dose of diamorphine. The nauseating effects of diamorphine can be helped by adding haloperidol or cyclizine to the infusion.

Nausea

This may be due to the disease process or the treatment. Haloperidol is probably the medication of choice,[10] in a dose of up to 10 mg over 24 hours. Alternatives are metoclopramide, cyclizine and the phenothiazines.

Causes of nausea such as constipation, hypercalcaemia, raised intracranial pressure and intestinal obstruction may be helped by symptomatic medication, but attention is also needed to the underlying cause.

Constipation

All terminally ill people are liable to constipation because of immobility and because constipation is a side-effect of all the stronger analgesic preparations. Even patients not eating need to void the cells sloughed off the bowel mucosa. Laxatives should be started as soon as strong opioids are prescribed.

Stimulant laxatives or stimulant plus softener are best. Senna and bisacodyl are good stimulants. Lactulose and ispaghula husk are good softeners. Docusate has both actions.

Constipation is a particularly trying symptom for the terminally ill. If no other way can be found, it is justified to use regular enemas to prevent constipation.

Diarrhoea

Faecal impaction is the commonest cause of diarrhoea in the terminally ill. Having excluded this, loperamide is probably the medication of choice.

Cough

Respiratory infections will cause cough and these may be treated with standard antibiotics. Even if the infection is secondary to bronchial obstruction by the neoplasm, treatment is the same. Cough due to wheeze may benefit from bronchodilators and steroids, but care must be taken not to provoke dyspepsia.

For cough without remediable cause, steam inhalers or nebulized saline or lignocaine can help loosen tacky secretions and provide relief. Simple linctus or codeine or pholcodine linctuses are also worth a try.

Mouth problems

Eighty per cent of patients with terminal cancer have xerostoma (a dry mouth), and in 75% of cases *Candida* is present.[12] Ice or pineapple chunks are helpful. *Candida* treatment with nystatin or amphotericin can be considered.

Patients who have a dry mouth as a result of radiotherapy or sicca syndrome can have artificial saliva products prescribed under Advisory Committee on Borderline Substances (ACBS) regulations. Suitable products are Glandosane and Salivix pastilles.

Depression

It is not unusual for terminally ill patients to become depressed, and this tendency is greater if other symptoms are not controlled. A process of psychological support needs to be started at the same time as the fatal diagnosis is made.

It is inappropriate to be optimistic about the long-term outcome in the terminally ill. Taking time to provide explanations of what is happening can demystify the illness and make it easier to come to terms with. It is also important to find out specifically if the patient has fears about dying. There is some evidence that death itself is quite without physical or emotional pain.[13] Patients can also be reassured that all possible efforts will be made to make sure that the terminal illness is as free of symptoms as possible.

Specific enquiries about symptoms may reveal problems which the patient 'did not want to trouble you' with. Good symptom control is important for the patient's psychological well-being.

If a clinical depression has occurred, then there is often a good response to standard antidepressant medication. Lesser degrees of depression respond less well to treatment. The fact that the depression is secondary to the terminal illness puts it very much in the reactive depression category, but the response to treatment depends more on severity of depressive symptoms rather than whether the depression is endogenous or reactive. People involved in long-term informal caring duties have poorer health than average. Depression may well feature in their reaction to the imminent death, and should be actively looked for. The maintenance of the caring team is an important function for the GP, and applies to lay carers as well as to the professionals.

Confusion

The cause of confusion may be the illness or the treatment. Haloperidol, diazepam, thioridazine, chlorpromazine and chlormethiazole may be considered in the disturbed or toxic patient.

Anorexia

Dietary advice may be needed. An appetizer, traditionally sherry, may be helpful. Small portions should be offered, and the patient should be tempted to eat rather than be bullied.

Liquid foods will be easier to take. If food is to be liquidized, it should be shown to the patient before it is processed so that some sense can be made of the uniformly brown pulp which the patient eventually gets to eat. Proprietary brands of liquid food are also available and these can be useful. A number of them can be prescribed under ACBS regulations for the malnutrition associated with chronic disease.

Sometimes steroids help to promote the appetite in a non-specific way. They do not, however, cause weight gain other than by fluid retention.[14]

Fungating tumours

The smell of a fungating tumour is a constant reminder of the inevitable. A course of metronidazole can be very useful to help mask the smell. Charcoal dressings or local radiotherapy to reduce tumour bulk are worth considering.

Respite care

Respite care for the terminally ill can be provided by hospitals or hospice (if available). The well-timed use of a respite admission may make all the difference between the carers' ability to cope or not.

Hospitals may only accept respite patients reluctantly. Such an attitude is inappropriate and short-sighted. A brief admission and a treatment evaluation, with attention to nutrition, fluid balance and skin care, will often reduce the subsequent need for acute care when the patient's state or the exhaustion of the carers provokes an emergency admission.

Hospices are charitable organizations. They will accept patients in an inpatient or day-patient basis, as well as providing terminal care advice (often through Macmillan nurses). The emphasis is on the active dimension of palliative care. More patients would wish to spend their terminal illness in a hospice rather than in hospital.

How well do we do? – Quality of care

Doctors tend to rate the severity of symptoms as less severe than their patients do. On the other hand, patients tend to rate their quality of life higher than their doctor's assessment.

Overall, 89% of patients and 91% of carers rate care as good or excellent. GPs and district nurses are rated as good by 71% of patients and family. Twenty-three per cent rate hospital services as poor, and less than half as good.[15]

When specific problems are addressed, the areas still causing concern to terminal patients and their families are:[4]

- Communication, especially at diagnosis.
- Coordination of services.
- Attitude of doctors.
- Delay in making the diagnosis.
- Problems persuading doctors to do home visits.
- Lack of financial advice.

It will be noticed that symptom control does not show on this list. In a 1992 MORI poll of terminally ill cancer sufferers, only 3% felt that they needed more prompt surgical care, but 24% felt in need of more counselling.[16] Now the problems over pain control are largely resolved, the next priority for the GP is to ensure that the patient and carers receive the necessary psychological support.

Benefits

Lack of advice about possible financial support is a common worry among the dying and their carers.

Attendance allowance

The Attendance Allowance is the benefit most often relevant to the terminal care situation. Eligible persons must be dependent on others for their bodily functions either by day, or by day and night. There is no means test. In order to qualify, the disability has to have been present for 6 months. This is clearly inappropriate in a terminal care situation and can be waived by use of the special rules provision where the GP fills in form DS 1500 attesting to the terminal nature of the illness.

The attendance allowance is not meant as a payment to the carers for their work. It is designed so that care can be bought in to help out and give the other carers a rest.

Invalid care allowance

The Invalid Care Allowance may be applied for if a carer has had to give up paid employment to fulfil caring duties.

In addition there are a number of national and local charities which may help with voluntary or paid carers, or the provision of equipment. The district nursing team will usually have a good idea of what is available locally.

Euthanasia

The law is quite clear. Killing people is against the law and attracts punishment. The situation where a patient dies as a side-effect of treating a disease or symptom is far less clear. Treatments primarily designed to combat serious symptoms, e.g. opiates, are widely used in terminal care, and the correct dose is that which controls the symptom. If this is a fatal dose, it is still unlikely to attract the interest of the constabulary. The intention, however, has to be symptom control, rather than to cause death.

The British Medical Association report on euthanasia[17] concluded that it wished euthanasia to remain illegal. However, the withholding of treatment from a terminally ill patient (for instance, antibiotics for end-stage chest infections) was regarded as acceptable. In practice a patient who is about to die is unlikely to respond to antibiotics anyway, which solves the dilemma.

In the Netherlands, a mechanism has been in place for some years to allow the termination of life by doctors when there is no chance of recovery, where symptoms are uncontrollable and where the patient asks for it. It is estimated that 2% of the deaths occurring in general practice are assisted in this way.[18]

The advance directive or living will is a mechanism by which people may express their feelings about life-salvaging treatments should they become terminally ill and mentally incompetent. The living will has no status in UK law, but a court decision in 1993 has indicated a possible change in the near future. It is already accepted as binding in some US states and elsewhere, where it works on the same principle as informed consent.[19]

References

1. Thorpe G. Enabling more dying people to remain at home. *Br Med J* 1993; **307**: 915–18
2. Townsend J, Frank AO, Fermont D *et al.* Terminal cancer care and patients' preferences for place of death. *Br Med J* 1990; **301**: 415–17
3. Griffith D. Respite care. *Br Med J* 1993; **306**: 160
4. Jones RVH, Hansford J and Fiske J. Death from cancer at home: the carers' perspective. *Br Med J* 1993; **306**: 249–51
5. Patient choice in managing cancer. *Drug Ther Bull* 1993; **31**: 77–79
6. McLauchlan CAJ. Handling distressed relatives and breaking bad news. *Br Med J* 1990; **301**: 1145–9
7. Brown A. The Macmillan service. *Med Dialogue* 1985; **40**
8. Finlay I and Forbes K. Symptom control in palliative care. *Update* 1994; **48**: 180–88
9. Haines A and Booroff A. Terminal care at home: perspectives in general practice. *Br Med J* 1986; **292**: 1051–3
10. Mersey Regional Drug Information Service and the Department of Pharmacology, University of Liverpool. Care of the dying. Drug information letter. *MeReC* 1991;
11. O'Neill WM. Pain in malignant disease. *Prescribers' J* 1993; **33**: 250–8
12. Jobins J, Bagg J, Finlay IG *et al.* Oral and dental disease in terminally ill patients. *Br Med J* 1992; **304**: 1612
13. Waine C. Terminal care. *R Coll GP Members' Reference Book* 1988; 176–80
14. Davis CL and Hardy JR. Palliative care. *Br Med J* 1994; **308**: 1359–62
15. Higginson I, Wade A and McCarthy M. Palliative care: views of patients and their families. *Br Med J* 1990; **301**: 277–81
16. *The Social Impact of Care in Great Britain*. London: MORI Health Research 1992
17. British Medical Association. *The Euthanasia Report*. London: BMA. 1988
18. Sheldon T. Euthanasia law does not end debate in the Netherlands. *Br Med J* 1993; **307**: 511–12
19. Davies J and Beresford D. The advance directive. *Med Defence Union J* 1991; **4**: 92–3

9

Behavioural problems in children

Aims

The trainee should:

- Be able to recognize normal childhood behaviour and the problems it might cause.
- Be aware of the more serious diagnostic possibilities which problem behaviour may indicate.
- Be able to give helpful advice to parents faced with problem behaviour, and to form collaborative links with the parents and other professionals whether or not the solution to the problem can be provided from primary care.

Preamble

The majority of children at least from time to time cause their parents and other carers anxiety. Problem behaviour is always a two-way process: the nature of the behaviour, and the response of the parents. Consequently parents always have to be involved in management. Care must be taken to ensure that problem behaviour is not regarded as the 'fault' of the parents. The cooperation of the parents is essential in all types of treatment.

On the other hand, some parents will tolerate very disruptive behaviour. This tolerance may give a significant insight into why the behaviour is occurring.

Behaviour must be seen in the context of the developmental age of the child. Selfish behaviour at the age of 2 is normal, but at 12 is unacceptable. This will often make problem behaviour at least understandable, if not tolerable. Stress or other illness may make a child retreat to a former developmental stage and so exhibit behaviour appropriate to that stage – so-called regression.

The GP and health visitor can often give advice on the appropriate management of minor behavioural problems. In rare instances, however, the behaviour is a result of a more severe problem. If there is any doubt about one of these more severe diagnoses, specialist assessment and help should be secured at an early stage.

The preschool child

All children are different. Even between siblings there may be major differences in temperament. Some authorities advocate the formal assessment of temperament using psychometric tests as a way of understanding behavioural traits.[1] Professionals and carers outside the family may be more aware of the range of normal behaviour seen in this age group, and be able to reassure the parents accordingly.[2]

Most problems in this age group can be tackled in primary care. Both parents need to be involved. In addition the health visitor can be an invaluable resource.

The preschool child is basically selfish, but this is quite normal. The need for attention is a primary one. The means used to achieve that attention are only abnormal if they are extreme.

This of course begs the question of why the child is resorting to such extreme methods. Issues to consider include:

- Is he or she receiving adequate attention?
- Has the available attention been attenuated by, for instance, a new sibling, or the mother getting a job?
- Has there been a significant loss of a relative or pet?
- Has there been a frightening experience?
- Is the behaviour the same in all circumstances, for instance does it also occur at granny's house?

The child who wishes more attention has four options for behavioural tactics which are outside parental control and cause sufficient disruption: temper tantrums, eating refusal, sleep refusal and refusal to defecate.

Temper tantrums

The usual age is 18 months to 3 years.[2] Tantrums are only effective if there is an audience. If the child is put in a safe place and left alone, and the tantrum not referred to again, then this method of getting attention rapidly loses its appeal.

Eating refusal

A child cannot be forced to eat. The behaviour causes extra parental anxiety as there is the additional concern that the poor eating will lead to ill health.

Weighing the child to demonstrate that no harm is resulting is a good way of alleviating anxiety. Very rarely there is a genuine and consistent failure to gain weight, and in such cases a more severe problem or even the extremely rare childhood example of anorexia nervosa should be remembered.

Sensible advice to parents includes:[2]

- Make mealtimes peaceful and free of tension. Wait till the siblings are at school.
- At first give small meals on a small plate.
- Parents and other family members should not comment on how little the child is eating.
- After reasonable encouragement, remove the meal and don't offer food till the next meal time.
- Make sure the child is receiving attention between meals in socially acceptable ways.

Bowel problems

A persisting refusal to defecate will result in a rectum packed with hard faeces, and any attempt at evacuation will then result in pain or even an anal fissure. In severe cases the rectum gets so distended that the reflex to evacuate is lost. Liquid faeces from higher up the colon may seep round the hard faeces and present as diarrhoea. This so-called spurious diarrhoea may be suspected in a child whose diarrhoea is preceded by a time of constipation.

Sometimes an enema is needed to break the log jam, followed by softening agents such as lactulose suspension. Underlying psychological stressors can be sought and dealt with at the same time.

Sleep problems

All children wake repeatedly through the night; the trick is to get them to go to sleep again without disturbing the household. Sleep problems often start around 2 years, which is just the time when the birth of a sibling is most likely, 2 years being a popular gap between babies. A problem with sleeping is the most common infant behavioural disorder presented to the GP.

Problems fall mainly into two categories:

Problems of going to bed and to sleep
This can usually be tackled by establishing a very definite bedtime routine. A sequence such as bath, then story, then drink, then cuddle, then to bed will establish the normality of going to sleep. It should be done at the same time each night. If bedtime needs to be brought forward, this can be done gradually, with bedtime getting 15 minutes earlier every 2 or 3 nights.

Problems of repeated waking
This is a commoner problem, with 10–20% of 3 year olds being affected. It is also more disruptive for the rest of the family. Some children wake up frightened; others wake and want to play: suitable responses should take account of these differences. There are two possible strategies – desensitizing and flooding.

1. In *desensitizing*, a regime is worked out which results in less time and attention with each successive disturbance. Each time the child cries, the parents wait for a slightly longer time before attending. Each attendance is slightly briefer than the one before.
2. In *flooding*, the child is left to cry, and is not attended at all. The neighbours need to be warned if this approach is being considered.

Other sleep problems are caused by *nightmares*, where the child wakes remembering the bad dream. These are usually self-limiting.
Night terrors happen during deeper sleep, and are not remembered. The child is distressed but still asleep and unresponsive. An older age group is involved, and problems may persist for years. The terrors often occur at the same time each night, so one useful strategy is to wake the child before the terror happens.

How to change a child's behaviour

Some principles underpin all the successful strategies for getting small children to change their habits. Because preschool children are essentially selfish, and because getting attention is a fundamental need, verbal and physical punishment rarely brings about the desired result. Friendly or angry attention is still attention.

• Set boundaries for acceptable behaviour. It's no good setting rules, then not sticking to them. If an exasperated parent backs down at the end of a prolonged bout of undesirable behaviour, this will convince the child that rules can indeed be broken, but only after a strenuous effort.

- Be consistent. Rules, when decided upon, should be adhered to. Other family members and carers must understand what the parents are trying to achieve and stick to the same rules.
- Penalties and punishments should be reasonable and brief. Any threats made should be achievable. The punishment should fit the crime.
- Reward good behaviour either by attention or by treats (of which star charts are surprisingly useful). Bad behaviour should be ignored if possible.

The junior school years

Behavioural problems in the 5–11 year olds are less common, but tend to be harder to deal with. In some cases the problem subsides spontaneously, but most need treatment. Difficulties are usually the result of wider pathology within the family, but occasionally because of significant pathology within the child.

It is estimated that 10% of children in this age group display behavioural problems, with more boys than girls being represented.[3] The more severe cases often go on to to be offenders in adult life. Global learning delay is often found to coexist.

What are the problems?

The behaviour of which the parents complain is usually an exaggeration of commonly found traits. The problem may be either one of degree, or of parental tolerance. The types of behaviour encountered may include:

- Disobedience, tantrums, occasional aggression and high levels of activity at home.
- Disruption in the classroom and aggression towards other children. There may be global learning disorders or particular problems with language.
- At age 6, children can usually distinguish between their property and that of others. Stealing and lying may be seen.
- Running away from home, engaging in dangerous activity, truancy.

Two other factors are particularly significant in this age group – somatization and hearing impairment.

Somatization
This is best defined as 'psychological distress giving rise to physical symptoms'.[4] About 10% of school-age children are affected, the commonest manifestations being headaches and abdominal pains. In about a fifth of the children seen in primary care there will be a psychological factor exacerbating the symptoms, and this rises to around a half of children attending general paediatric hospital clinics.[4]

Of those children referred to a specialist because of abdominal pain, only 5% turn out to have a serious cause for the pain. It is, however, necessary to rule out physical pathology before family anxiety can be relieved and a psychological diagnosis agreed. A discussion of the physical effects of psychological illness and teasing out the possible sources of stress from the history can both be useful ways of making progress with the child and family.

Children with recurrent abdominal pains tend to be conformist, eager to gain approval, and with a sensitivity to distress and insecurity. There has often been a recent excess of significant life events, such as deaths, exams, etc. Somatization disorders in parents are associated with an excess of unexplained physical disorders in their children.[4]

The overall health of the child will reassure the GP that a serious physical diagnosis is not being missed. Using a diagnosis like 'abdominal migraine' may actually be true, and if not, at least serves to emphasize the non-serious nature of the pain. The majority of children do improve with time, with a reduction in the frequency of the attacks, and either a reduction in severity or a reduction in the alarm caused by the pain.

An explanation of the disorder should be helpful and make the symptoms less worrying to child and parents. Specific stress management techniques may help, but these are probably best left to the child psychiatry services.

A recent sudden onset of a psychosomatic disorder may indicate sexual abuse.

Symptoms may also get tied up in school refusal problems.

Hearing loss
Sensorineural hearing loss in children is rare and usually congenital. The usual cause of conductive loss is secretory otitis media (glue ear) and it is estimated that up to 80% of children have at least one episode of this in their lives.[5]

Glue ear is commoner in boys and peaks at 3–6 years. Hearing loss is often the only symptom, and is commonly suspected at first by the parents. If the parents report concern about their child's hearing, this should be taken very seriously, whatever the lack of other evidence to support the diagnosis.

Hearing loss causes the child perceptual and expressive problems. The inability to take in information accurately leads to confusion, frustration and anger. The child who is unable to hear instructions is unable to please his or her parents and so fails to gain approval. Alternative behavioural means are found in order to elicit a response.

Expressive problems are caused by the poor development of language, which is a consequence of not being able to hear others speak. Non-verbal communication is therefore attempted, and so behavioural changes result.

Up to half of children with hearing deficit will display behavioural problems.[5] Those most frequently seen are over-activity, short attention span, poor relations with other children, temper tantrums and being out of parental control. Longer-term problems include conduct disorders which last to adolescence, subtle language deficits, poorer educational attainment, persisting difficulties with relationships, and long-term effects on self-esteem and self-confidence.

Audiometry is an accurate and non-invasive procedure. Any child in whom there is suspicion of a hearing deficit, especially if there are behavioural problems, should be properly tested.

What is the GP's role?

The child's GP is in a unique position to help with behavioural problems because of ongoing knowledge of the child and particularly of the other members of the family. Time should be spent at the outset to establish the facts of each case, and even if the child is referred on for specialist care, it is appropriate to maintain contact to support the family. Liaison with the health visitor will ensure a consistency of approach, and also give further insights.

What are the symptoms?
Details of the problem behaviour should be sought. An A, B, C analysis can be useful – what are the antecedents? Of what nature is the behaviour? What are the consequences? Does the behaviour happen in all circumstances, or only at home or at school? Are there any learning difficulties coexisting? Is there an abnormally short attention span?

How do the parents react?
The parents may have their own problems causing inability to cope, for instance depression or learning difficulties. There may be poor support from relatives and friends, particularly in single-parent households. Parental tolerance may be lower than average: they may over-react to some types of behaviour, such as aggression, or they may have formed their expectations of behaviour from an older child who has a different temperament.

How hard are the parents willing to work to bring about the behavioural change? Their cooperation is vital for success.

Are there family stresses?
Strains within the marriage may cause, or indeed be the consequence of, difficult child behaviour. Some families lack appropriate parenting skills with respect to giving the child attention and reacting to problem behaviour. There may have been a separation or death in the family, to which everyone is reacting.

What are the home circumstances?
Problem behaviour is commoner in overcrowded and deprived households. There may be insufficient space and toys for play. Play may not be adequately supervised. There may be too much or too little contact with adults and other children.

Could anything more serious be going on?
Rarely, one of the more severe problems mentioned below may be present. It is also appropriate to be aware of the behavioural consequences of physical or sexual abuse. Occasionally, physical illnesses are present, such as diabetes, thyroid disease, etc.

Problem behaviour is by no means always produced by adverse circumstances. However, any possible problem identified should be noted, as this may indicate what sort of therapeutic intervention might be appropriate.

More serious problems

A number of serious pathologies may rarely come to light at this age. The GP should maintain a suspicion for these. Parents will often fear a serious cause for their child's behaviour, so the GP should at least have an idea of how to rule out major problems.

Hyperactivity
The term hyperactivity can be overused as a label for any

boisterous behaviour with which parents have difficulty coping. This is not helped, as there is no agreed definition, so that in the USA the definition used is rather laxer than in the UK, with the corresponding increase in numbers diagnosed. Using UK criteria, about 1 child in 500 is affected, and most cases are identified before the age of 6.[6]

Getting a good history is more important than the 'snapshot' impression gained during a surgery visit, which may be influenced by the child's tiredness, boredom or intercurrent illness. The story will be of a child in constant motion, settling neither to desk nor table. Objects and toys are handled then quickly discarded, without play or activity being sustained. Books and television are looked at only briefly.

Social skills with adults and children are poor so the child has few friends. There may be risk-taking, opposition to rules, aggressive and destructive behaviour. Levels of activity are always high, and there is less than average sleep, but disturbance at night is unusual.

A number of authors, in particular Feingold in the USA,[13] have written extensively on the possible dietary causes of hyperactivity. So considerable has been the influence of this writing that most parents will have tried to exclude additives from their child's diet before presenting to the GP. Except in a very few cases, there is little convincing evidence that particular foods or additives have an influence on hyperactivity.[7]

Autism

Autism is a developmental disorder probably brought on by organic brain damage in early years.[8] It is of unknown origin but is not caused by emotional trauma or poor parenting.

Around 5 per 10 000 are severely affected, and a further 20 per 10 000 have autistic tendencies. It is a rare disorder which the average GP will see only once every 80 years.

Autism often accompanies other developmental disorders, and four boys are affected for every girl. Of those diagnosed, 10% will be able to live independently, 30% will need some support, and the rest will be significantly handicapped and completely dependent.

Diagnosis is usually made by age 3. Parental observations are of greatest importance. The role of the GP is to be suspicious and refer on for proper assessment.

Important symptoms are:[9]

- Showing what they want by using an adult's hand.
- Parroting a question instead of answering it.
- Laughing or giggling, often for no reason.

- Talking incessantly about one topic.
- Exhibiting bizarre behaviour.
- Handling or spinning objects.
- Avoiding eye contact.
- Avoiding creative play but ordering objects repetitively.
- Joining in games with other children only if adults insist.
- Doing tasks that do not involve social interaction quickly.

Dyslexia

Dyslexia is a severe difficulty with learning to read, spell and write, despite average or above-average intelligence and normal schooling. A subgroup have specific difficulty with spelling – dysgraphia. Other problems may be an inability to read music or difficulty with mathematics.

Some 4–10% of children are affected, depending on the diagnostic criteria used.[10] Four boys are affected for each girl. There is evidence of genetic transmission.

The signs of dyslexia include:

- Late speech development.
- Difficulty labelling known objects or people's names.
- Persistent word searching.
- Excessive spoonerisms.
- Difficulty learning nursery rhymes, days of the week, months of the year, etc.
- Often clumsy.
- Difficulty throwing, catching or kicking a ball, or with hopping, skipping and clapping rhythms.
- Late learning to fasten buttons.
- Continuing to put shoes on the wrong feet in spite of the discomfort.

If dyslexia is suspected, the job of the GP is to refer on to an educational psychologist for full assessment and management. Treatment is by special educational techniques. The sooner the condition is recognized and treatment begun, the less disruption is caused to the child's development.

School refusal

On any one day, 10% of children are absent from school, but only 1 or 2% are away because of school refusal.[11] School attendance is required by the Education Act 1981, and the Children Act 1989 contains powers to supervise the child whose school attendance is poor.

It is not unusual for school refusal to present as physical symptoms with no obvious cause. Typical somatized symptoms include:

- Nausea.
- Abdominal pain.
- Headache.
- 'Wobbly legs'.

There are four categories of children who do not attend school:

1. School refusal proper is where the child resists all parental efforts to get him or her to school. It is likely to be a continuing problem.
2. Truancy is when the child misses school without the knowledge of the carers. It tends to be a group activity.
3. School phobia is when the child is overwhelmingly frightened of some aspect of the school, and so will not attend.
4. Withholding is where the parents collude to keep the child from school. The parents may want the child at home either because of fears over the child's health, or because of their own psychological needs.

Having established the facts, the GP will wish to involve the teacher and educational welfare officer, and possibly the educational psychologist. It is usually appropriate to organize a gentle graduated re-exposure to the school environment. Flooding does not usually work.

Adolescence

What is normal?

The Isle of Wight study into the psychiatric health of 14 and 15 year olds found an incidence of psychiatric disorder of 20%, a figure similar to that found in adults, but greater than the 7% found in children. In the same survey, 40% of adolescents reported that they had felt so miserable that they had cried, and 20% had had feelings of self deprecation.[12]

Adolescence is a time of great change and emotions of unparalleled intensity. Most survive the process intact without alienating their families,[12] but the upheavals along the way can be considerable.

As well as the bodily and life changes which are occurring, there is a tension between the desire for autonomy – individuation – and the loss of the security of the child's role within the family – separation.

Adolescence is also a time when a desire for reliable information from an impartial source is very strong. Twenty-five per cent of adolescents regard the GP as a suitable authority for involvement with their problems.

As with the younger ages, behaviour only becomes a problem when it gets to an unacceptable level. The ability of the adolescent to cause disruption is greater because of greater physical strength and social knowledge.

The reasons for difficulties in adolescents are:

• The normal process of growing up.
• Persisting childhood problems.
• Reaction to a stressor.
• Psychiatric disorder.

Types of problem

Emotional
With all the pressures of rapid change and turmoil, it's not surprising that emotional problems arise. Misery is quite common, and this is the most likely age for parasuicide to occur. Suicide proper is relatively rare, but getting commoner. Anxiety, phobias and obsessive/compulsive disorder may occur.

Sexual
Sexual doubt and experimentation are common. Surveys suggest that adolescents are not as sexually promiscuous as the tabloid headlines would have us believe, but this does not usually reassure parents. Some adolescents do involve themselves in unsafe sexual practices, often as a means of asserting independence, or of achieving peer approval.

Eating
Dieting is almost universal among adolescent girls, and in up to 3% of 16 year olds an eating disorder is present.[12] Obesity is associated with low self-esteem, and is also a risk factor for bulimia nervosa.

School
Varieties of school non-attendance are commoner when the child is changing schools, when separation problems may re-emerge. Disruption in class and poor achievement often coexist. Later on,

poor job prospects may provoke the feeling that school isn't worth the effort.

Family
The struggle for adulthood may be thwarted by the traditional family authority structure.

Trouble with the police
Delinquency may be viewed as an extension of risk-taking behaviour, a desire to beat authority, or an attempt to promote status among the peer group. Most delinquent behaviour does not lead to offending in later life.

Substance abuse
The commonest drugs used are alcohol, solvents and cannabis, and much abuse never extends beyond the experimental stage. The possibility of drug abuse should be borne in mind when parents describe a recent personality change.

Psychiatric disorders
Just occasionally the early stages of schizophrenia will present as a behavioural disorder. The signs at this early stage are usually florid, with hallucinations well to the fore.

What can the GP do?

At a minimum, the GP should spend enough time to clarify the facts, and find out who is most concerned by the behaviour. Some problem behaviour may in fact be normal, and this can be discussed with the parents.

The more interested GP will set up a series of interviews with the child and family together and separately. It usually requires a particular effort to hear the child's side of things, especially if he or she is suspicious and sees you as on the parents' side.

Many child psychiatry units operate as a team involving not only psychiatrists, but also psychologists, specialized community psychiatric nurses, and the more esoteric practitioners such as dance and art therapists. They are probably in the best position to arrange the assessment and treatment of cases.

References

1. Oberllaid F. The clinical assessment of temperament in infants and young children. *Maternal Child Health* 1991; **16**: 1417

2. Cook N. Behaviour problems. *The Practitioner* 1993; **237**: 687–91
3. McColl M. Behavioural problems in childhood. *Med Monitor* 1991; **4**: 46–7
4. Garralda ME and Hughes TP. Worried sick – somatisation in children. *Maternal Child Health* 1994; 40–4
5. Barber W., Griffiths MV and Williams R. Behaviour disorders and hearing loss in preschool children. *Update* 1992; **44**: 1132–40
6. McColl M. Managing hyperactive children. *Med Monitor* 1992; **5**: 65–9
7. Taylor E and Heptinstall E. Dietary treatment for hyperactivity – does it work? *Maternal Child Health* 1990; **15**: 98–102
8. Plachta J. Be vigilant over bizarre behaviour. *GP Newspaper*. May 8 1992; pp 66–67
9. *Aids to Diagnosis of Autism*. London: National Autistic Society. 1992
10. Goulandris N., Newton A. and Auger J. Dyslexia. *GP Newspaper* Decmber 4 1992; 43–8
11. McColl M. Children who won't go to school. *Med Monitor* 1992; **5**:
12. Lewin C. and Williams R. Difficult adolescents. *Update* 1992; **45**: 333–9
13. Feingold BF. Hyperkinesis and learning disabilities linked to artificial food flavours and colours. *Am J Nurs* 1975; **75**: 797–803

The menopause and hormone replacement therapy (HRT)

Aims

The trainee should:

- Be able to counsel a woman presenting with climacteric symptoms.
- Be able to assess the individual suitability of a patient for HRT.
- Have knowledge of the use of HRT in general practice, and be able to describe a care plan for a patient on HRT.

What is the menopause?

The menopause is the time of life when the periods have ceased. The mean age when women in the UK have their last period is 50 years ± 1½ years.[1] There is a broad range so that 1% of women will have ceased periods by the age of 40, and 1% will not have their last period till age 58.

It is not clear why the menopause occurs, as there is an interplay of racial, nutritional, socioeconomic and familial factors. For the 5–10 years before the menopause there is a gradual decrease in fertility as anovulatory periods become commoner, so the failure in ovarian function is gradual.[1]

What is the climacteric?

The climacteric is the cessation of the periods and also all the symptoms surrounding this event. Most women are delighted that their periods have stopped, and it is the associated symptoms which cause all the trouble.

The climacteric has been associated with a wide variety of symptoms including hot flushes, sweats, palpitations, dizziness, insomnia, apprehension, depression, headache, lost libido, bone and joint pain, urge incontinence.[2] The symptoms which are demonstrably due to lack of oestrogen are vasomotor instability (which occurs in 50–75% of perimenopausal women),[1] and atrophy of oestrogen-dependent tissues such as the vagina, urethra and trigone.

The psychological symptoms of the climacteric are more difficult to correlate with oestrogen deficiency. Social circumstances and life events are better at predicting their occurrence than are oestrogen levels.[2]

In addition, there is a cultural component to women's experiences of the climacteric. The reporting of vasomotor symptoms in some parts of the world is very low. In the Japanese language there is no word for 'hot flush'.[2]

What causes climacteric symptoms?

The climacteric occurs at a time when there are likely to be other major changes occurring in the woman's life. The loss of fertility may be a cause of sadness. Existing children are often at the difficult adolescent stage. The marital relationship may be not be standing up to the test of time. The career may be stagnating as the woman has reached the peak of her abilities. These factors will confound the effects of oestrogen deficiency.

Research into the climacteric has looked at the effects of oestrogen supplements on the symptoms, with the assumption that if the symptom is relieved, then that symptom must be caused by oestrogen deficiency. However, the oestrogens used in the supplements are either synthetic or animal products, and so are unlike the woman's own oestrogen. The attention paid by the researcher to the woman may also have an influence on the severity of the symptoms.

The surveys done generally show a considerable placebo response to therapy. The benefits of oestrogen in terms of overall well-being seem to outweigh the improvement in specific symptoms.[2]

The population which ends up on prolonged HRT is different in a number of respects from the general population. Women on HRT tend to eat healthier diets, take more exercise and have more contacts with their GP than women who decide not to stay on HRT.[3]

It is now possible to measure with some confidence the effect of HRT on some important disease processes, notably breast and gynaecological cancers, strokes, heart attacks and osteoporosis. As far as research is concerned, these represent 'hard' end-points. The 'soft' end-points such as psychological well-being are harder to quantify reliably.

Which women ask for HRT?

Around 90% of perimenopausal women are aware of HRT, mainly through the mass media,[4] and over half are aware of its use in preventing osteoporosis.[5] Around 10% know of the benefits in the prevention of stroke and heart attacks.[4] Despite this, most users of HRT do so because of symptoms such as hot flushes, vaginal dryness, mood changes and lack of energy.[5]

Around half of perimenopausal women are not troubled by symptoms to any significant degree. It appears that women who request HRT are more likely to regard the climacteric as a deficiency disorder rather than a natural and inevitable part of getting older.[5]

About 10% of eligible women take HRT.[6]

Which women would benefit from HRT?

There are two indications for postmenopausal HRT: treatment of symptoms of oestrogen deficiency, and prevention of long-term complications such as osteoporosis and cardiovascular disease.

Osteoporosis

Women at particular risk of osteoporosis should be offered HRT. There is no completely reliable way of making an assessment of risk as, for instance, 30% of bone mass may be lost before X-ray changes are apparent,[7] and the predictive value of bone densimetry is not proven.[3] Some features may, however, make osteoporosis more likely:[3]

- Early menopause or an episode of premenopausal amenorrhoea. Whether the menopause is natural or as a result of surgery does not seem to matter. After oophorectomy the oestrogen deficit is immediate, and after hysterectomy ovarian function ceases within the next 3 years.[7]
- Women who are thin and have a slight frame.
- Women who smoke cigarettes.
- Women who have a family history of osteoporosis.
- Women who have recently been treated with glucocorticoids.

Cardiovascular

There are clear benefits from unopposed oestrogen treatment in the reduction of cardiovascular events, but the addition of progestagen (as is usually the case) may abolish this benefit. On current evidence it is better to concentrate on the other factors involved in cardiovascular disease, such as smoking, rather than use HRT.[3]

Who should not have HRT?

Contraindications to HRT are few:

- Undiagnosed vaginal bleeding either before or during HRT should be investigated.
- Endometrial cancer or hyperplasia is usually considered a contraindication, but there is no evidence that, following a radical cure, the use of HRT worsens the prognosis.[3]
- A history of breast cancer usually precludes HRT, but some authorities are prepared to use hormones in the severely symptomatic patient who is fully informed as to the risks and benefits of treatment.
- HRT does not increase the chance of venous thrombosis.[3] Spurious contraindications have been used in the past to deny women HRT. They include hyperlipidaemia, hypertension, diabetes and impending elective surgery.

Why do most women stop taking HRT?

Overall only a small minority of eligible women take HRT. Even after specific teaching about the risks of osteoporosis, only around 20% of women will begin treatment,[5] and only 30% of women who are at particular risk because they have had a bilateral oophorectomy are likely to be persuaded to embark on treatment.[5]

Of those women who do begin treatment, between 30 and 60% stop within a few weeks or months, often without seeing their doctor first.[6] A number of reasons have been postulated for this behaviour:

- Eighty per cent of women on HRT have periods, and this is seen as the most unwelcome side-effect. In one survey, 15% of the women said they would be prepared to have a hysterectomy rather than suffer the restart of their menses.[5]

- Sixty per cent of women are worried about the long-term effects of treatment, in particular cancer and weight gain.[5]
- Many GPs have only patchy knowledge of the risks and benefits of HRT, and are motivated more by 'intuition and general philosophical considerations rather than a formal appraisal of likely risks versus benefits'.[8]
- Doctors may try to offer advice rather than opinions when counselling women about the possible use of HRT. This can be perceived by the patient as the doctor being unenthusiastic about the treatment. Since doctor recommendation is a powerful motivator, this perceived reluctance has a negative effect.[5]
- Some doctors are put off using HRT by their experiences with the combined oral contraceptive pill (COP). The doses of hormone used in HRT are much smaller, and the oestrogens used are different. An exaggerated perception of the dangers of the COP may have been developed when larger-dose products were the norm.

What are the risks and benefits of HRT?

The GP will often be asked for an opinion by patients who would like to know whether HRT would help them.

Research into the effects of HRT have been dogged by a number of methodological problems. Surveys have used different hormone regimes for different periods of time. Some populations have been hospital-based, some clinic-based and some general practice-based. Many studies have been observational and retrospective rather than prospective. When looking at the risks and benefits, many surveys have used 'surrogate' end-points for disease – in particular, changes in lipid profile have been used as a proxy for ischaemic heart disease and coronary deaths.

Notwithstanding these reservations, it is possible to form some conclusions:

Cardiovascular disease

Most of the research has been done with oral unopposed conjugated oestrogen, and this shows a clear improvement in fatal and non-fatal heart attack of up to 45%, and a 15% reduction in stroke.[3] The value of patches is not proven. Progestagens adversely affect lipid profiles and so the protective effect of opposed oestrogen is unproven.

Osteoporosis

Hip fractures cost £500m per year (1991), and carry a 20% 6-month mortality: 50% of survivors lose independence and need long-term care.[7] HRT reduces the risk of hip fracture by 50–75% after 5 years' use of both opposed and unopposed oestrogen.[3] The risk of a vertebral fracture is reduced by 75–80% by using HRT.[3]

Bone loss resumes as soon as HRT is stopped, so the intention is to delay bone loss so that fracture is unlikely before death. The median age for hip fracture is 75 years, so causing a delay in bone loss of 5–10 years is sufficient to secure benefit. Old ladies get fractures because they fall over: cognitive impairment is also a risk factor for fractures.

Cancer

Cancer of the breast is 1.3 times more likely after 10 years of HRT.[3] Cancer of the endometrium is 10 times more likely after 10 years of HRT: this risk is virtually abolished by opposing with progestagen for 12 days per month.

Risk : benefit overview

It has been estimated[9] that if 100 000 menopausal women aged 50–75 were treated with *unopposed oestrogen*, then the changes in mortality would be:

- Osteoporosis 563 lives saved.
- Gallbladder disease 2 lives lost.
- Endometrial cancer 63 lives lost.
- Breast cancer 187 lives lost.
- Heart attack 5250 lives saved.

The total reduction in mortality is thus 5561 lives or 41% of the total expected mortality. It should be remembered, however, that most women on HRT also take progestagens, and the risks and benefits of this dual treatment may well be different.

Does HRT work for climacteric symptoms?

A study of over 3000 women attending a special menopause clinic reported in 1988.[2] The cohort was in many respects not representative of the population as a whole; for instance, there were twice as many social class I and II women.

Ninety per cent reported feeling better when using HRT, but the improvement of specific symptoms was far less compelling. Of 25 symptoms enquired about, only vasomotor symptoms (41%), general well-being (28%), depression, anxiety and tension (16%), sexual and vaginal factors (13%), and ability to cope (12%), were mentioned as being improved by more than 10% of respondents.

Information about HRT came mainly from the media and friends (48%), and health professionals (41%). Twenty per cent felt that they had exerted pressure on their GP to start HRT.

Oral and parenteral sources of oestrogen are equally effective in controlling the symptoms of oestrogen deficit.[3]

How do you start HRT?

If periods have ceased and there are climacteric symptoms, then the diagnosis is not in doubt. Following hysterectomy, however, it may be necessary to measure serum follicle-stimulating hormone levels. A result of over 20 u/l confirms the diagnosis.

Since compliance with HRT is such a problem, it is important that as much information as possible is shared with the patient. If the woman is unlikely to use the treatment for any reason, it is as well to know this from the outset.

Issues to be discussed[6]

It is important that women proposing to take HRT should have sufficient information in order to make an informed decision. Compliance is more likely if the woman knows what she's letting herself in for. Discussion can be reinforced by written material. Some women benefit from being referred to specialist menopausal clinics for their care.

- *The menopause* – what hormones are, why the menopause occurs, and what the consequences are of oestrogen deficiency.
- *HRT* – what HRT is and how it works, what it can and cannot do, and what the short- and long-term benefits are.
- *Formulations* – the range, dosages and routes of delivery, and the importance of progestagens.
- *Safety* – the dose is lower than the amount the premenopausal woman makes herself. The risk of breast cancer over 10 years' use, the negligible risk of endometrial cancer if progestagens are used, and the low risk of thrombosis and hypertension if natural oestrogen is used.

- *Side-effects* – Therapy can be tailored to minimize side-effects. Oestrogenic effects usually settle and therapy does not cause weight gain.
- Monitoring programme required while on treatment.
- Duration of treatment.

The physical examination[10]

Having observed the contraindications to HRT, a baseline of physical examination is required:

1. Pelvic examination if this has not been done in the previous 12 months.
2. Breast palpation if not done in the previous 12 months.
3. Cervical smear if not done in the previous 3 years.
4. Mammography if not done in the previous 3 years.
5. Blood pressure.[11]
6. Urine dipstick for protein.[11]

What should be prescribed?

Continuous oral treatment with conjugated oestrogen is recommended.[3] The oestrogen should be opposed by progestagen for 12 days of each 4-week cycle if the uterus is intact, even if there has been an endometrial ablation procedure. Since two types of tablet are included in HRT, two prescription charges are levied.

Conjugated oestrogens are described as natural to distinguish them from the manufactured synthetic variety which seems to have a greater thrombotic potential. However, these natural hormones are extracted from horse urine, so they are only natural for horses.

Patches can be used if tablets cause a problem. They have theoretical advantages over oral treatment because the first pass through the liver is avoided, but whether this leads to clinical benefit is unproven.[3] It is likely that patches will bring about the same benefits as oral treatment, but this too is unproven. Twenty per cent of users will develop a rash because of the plaster.[10] Until a recent product was developed which includes a progestagen patch, it was necessary for users still to use progestagens in tablet form.

Oestrogen implants last for 6 months and can bring about high levels of oestrogen. They have to be inserted surgically, and in the woman with a uterus, progestagens in tablet form still have to be taken. In some women a tolerance develops so that the implants have to be given at decreasing intervals because of the return of symptoms, even though the serum oestrogen levels are above physiological.

What are the side-effects of HRT?

Oestrogens can cause breast and sometimes epigastric tenderness. Reducing the dose often helps. Progestagens cause more problems, and this may limit compliance. Breast tenderness, bloatedness, abdominal cramps, depression, anxiety and irritability are all described. Changing the progestagen may help.

Up to 80% of women on HRT have withdrawal bleeds. Fertility is not restored. Since the return of periods is a major reason why women do not start or do not continue taking HRT, a number of strategies have been tried to abolish this side-effect.

Tibolone possesses weak oestrogenic, progestational and androgenic properties. It will reduce menopausal symptoms and helps to reduce bone loss. Periods are much less likely, but bleeding may still occur and so tibolone should not be used in the first postmenopausal year.

Continuous progestagen can be used with the oestrogen, and after a year's use, 95% of women will be amenorrhoeic.[12] However, the progestagen is more likely to cause side-effects, so compliance may be a problem. A 35% drop-out rate can be expected.

What follow-up of patients on HRT is required?

A woman on HRT should be seen every 3–6 months. Side-effects should be enquired after, in particular weight changes, abdominal pains and breast swellings or discomfort. Any unscheduled bleeds at any stage in therapy should be investigated. Unlike the COP, bleeds occur at the start of a packet of tablets, and not before the next packet begins.

Blood pressure should be checked, and encouragement given to self-examine the breasts. The need for mammography and cervical cytology is the same as for women not taking HRT.

For women on HRT because of climacteric symptoms, it is appropriate to review at each attendance whether or not the HRT can be discontinued. If symptoms are completely abolished, the HRT can be stopped, but resumed if symptoms return.

What about those who cannot or will not use HRT?

Vasomotor symptoms

It is important to establish that the flushes are menopausal. Panic attacks, drug reactions (nifedipine, isosorbide) and carcinoid can all cause flushing.

Clonidine has been shown in some – but not all – trials to be helpful for flushes. The mode of action is not clear.

β-Blockers do not help flushes but are effective for associated symptoms of anxiety and tachycardia.

Pyridoxine is used to prevent flushes but research evidence for its efficacy is lacking.[13]

Osteoporosis

Regular exercise reduces hip fractures by 50% and stopping smoking reduces hip fractures by 25%.[3] A diet containing at least 1000 mg of calcium a day is recommended,[11] and a few minutes' exposure to daylight each day is sufficient to stimulate vitamin D formation. Heavy alcohol consumption is to be discouraged.

Established osteoporosis can be treated with other agents such as etidronate, stanazol, progestagens alone or calcitonin.

Coronary heart disease

There is insufficient evidence to support the routine use of HRT for the prevention of cardiovascular disease. Other well-recognized risk factors such as smoking, lack of exercise and poor diet should be addressed.

How long should HRT continue?

Vasomotor symptoms

For vasomotor symptoms, treatment need only go on as long as symptoms are troublesome. There is a tendency for symptoms to resolve over the course of time, so it is reasonable to stop treatment every 6 months to see if symptoms have settled.

Other climacteric symptoms

For other symptoms of the climacteric, treatment may be continued as long as it seems to help. The use of HRT seems to do more good than harm, even in those at low risk of oestrogen deficiency conditions. It is worth at each review asking about whether the treatment is still required.

Osteoporosis

The aim of using HRT to prevent the problems caused by osteoporosis is to delay bone loss until such time as the patient is likely to have died before there is a substantial risk of an osteoporotic fracture. In practical terms, 10 years of treatment will delay the usual peak age for fractures – about 75 – until 85, which is beyond the average life expectancy.

When stopping HRT, it is best to halve the oestrogen dose at first, keeping the progestagen unchanged. Later, treatment can be ceased completely.[11]

References

1. Scott A and Crowder AM. Menopause. *Update* 1993; **47**: 536–41
2. Hunt K. Perceived value of treatment among a group of long-term users of hormone replacement therapy. *Br J Gen Pract* 1988; **38**: 398–401
3. Jacobs HS and Loeffler FE. Postmenopausal hormone replacement therapy. *Br Med J* 1992; **305**: 1403–8
4. Kadri AZ. Hormone replacement therapy – a survey of perimenopausal women in a community setting. *Br J Gen Pract* 1991; **41**: 109–12
5. Kadri AZ. Women's attitudes regarding hormone replacement therapy at the menopause. RCGP Members' Reference Book 1992; 225–9
6. MacPherson S. Women drop HRT because of myths. *GP Newspaper* June 9 1994;
7. Dixon AStJ. *Osteoporosis and the Family Doctor. Reports on Rheumatic Diseases.* London: Arthritis and Rheumatism Council. 1991
8. Goddard MK. Hormone replacement therapy and breast cancer, endometrial cancer and cardiovascular disease: risks and benefits. *Br J Gen Pract* 1992; **42**: 120–5
9. Sturdee D. Hormone replacement therapy: risks and benefits. *Practitioner* 1990; **234**: 471–4
10. Garnett TJ and Studd JWW. Monitoring hormone replacement therapy in general practice. *Update* 1992; **45**: 426–30
11. Coope J. Managing menopausal problems in general practice. *RCGP Connection* 1991; **41**: 10–11
12. Holland N and Studd J. Wider applications for oestrogen replacement therapy. *J Sexual Health* 1993; **20**: 200–3
13. Van Schaick S. Symptomatic treatment of hot flushes. *Update* 1993; **46**: 61–65

Current issues in preconceptual and antenatal care

Aims

The trainee should:

- Be able to counsel the woman who attends for preconceptual advice.
- Be able to advise the pregnant woman on matters likely to secure the best pregnancy outcome.
- Be able to express such advice in terms readily accessible to the patient.

Preamble

Nothing grips the public imagination and the popular press like a baby story. Hazards which may cause damage to unborn babies have a particular fascination, and readily come to public attention. Many GPs will have had the experience of being consulted by an anxious potential parent concerned over some new information that has appeared in the media.

Reliable evidence on these very topical issues is often lacking as the news hits the press well before it appears in the medical journals. Good information takes time to gather, and will always be incomplete as it is ethically impossible to do randomized trials on pregnant women. This is also the case with the use of medication in pregnancy. If a pregnant woman is invited to take a new drug to see if it will damage her baby, her likely response is not in doubt.

This chapter is a review, with evidence, of some of the issues which have been discussed over the past 5 years.

Antenatal vitamins

Vitamin A

There have been no cases in the UK, but reports from abroad indicate that it is prudent not to overdose on vitamin A during pregnancy because of the risk of fetal abnormality. Most of the few cases reported from the rest of the world were associated with excessive vitamin A supplements being consumed, and in only one case has a large daily intake of liver been implicated.

Recommended doses of vitamin A in the UK are 750 µg/day normally, and 1200 µg during lactation. A daily maximum of 3000 µg is suggested.[1]

Recommendations
- Women who are pregnant or intending to become pregnant should be careful of dosages when taking vitamin supplements which contain vitamin A.
- A portion of liver contains four to 12 times the recommended daily dosage for a pregnant woman. Liver and liver products such as liver pâté and liver sausage should be avoided.
- Sufficient vitamin A can be found in other foods such as dairy products, green vegetables, margarine, eggs, carrots, tomatoes and fruit.

Folic acid

The link between neural tube defects and folic acid deficit has been suspected for some time. The issue was clarified by 1991, and specific recommendations were circulated by the Department of Health.[2]

The amount of folic acid needed from before conception until the 12th week of pregnancy is 0.4 mg/day. This regime will minimize the risk of a neural tube defect.

Recommendations
Preventing first occurrence   Women are advised to increase their intake of foods rich in folic acid, such as vegetables (particularly sprouts), fruit and cereals, especially where fortified with folate. In addition, a vitamin tablet with 0.4 mg folate should be taken.

Preventing recurrence A supplement of 4 or 5 mg should be taken daily before and during the first 12 weeks of pregnancy.

Antenatal infections

Chickenpox

Only 2% of chickenpox occurs in patients over 20 years old, but this group contributes 25% of all deaths from the disease, usually because of varicella pneumonia. The immunocompromised are more at risk, and the mild immunosuppression associated with pregnancy may contribute to the often quoted but not proven view that the pregnant are more at risk from the complications of chickenpox.[3]

Rarely, fetal death or premature labour is caused, but this reflects the severity of the illness rather than the chickenpox as such.

A syndrome of fetal infection was first described in 1947. The characteristic feature is hypoplasia of a single limb, with skin lesions in a dermatome distribution on the same limb. Other described features include hydrocephalus, microcephaly, eye problems, gastrointestinal and urogenital structural problems, and growth retardation.

The risk of fetal varicella syndrome after maternal varicella in the first trimester is 3% (but compare this with the risk of a significant abnormality in all pregnancies of 2.3%). Infection in later pregnancy rarely causes congenital abnormality. However, after infection in late pregnancy, 20–60% of the consequent neonates get chickenpox within a few days of birth, with a mortality of up to 30%.

Recommendations
- In the susceptible pregnant woman with good evidence of chickenpox contact, zoster immune globulin should be given within 4 days of contact.
- Zoster immune globulin should be given to infants who develop chickenpox at or just after birth.
- Severe or progressive maternal or neonatal chickenpox should be treated with intravenous acyclovir.

Toxoplasmosis

This is caused by a small protozoan, *Toxoplasma gondii*, which is endemic in this country. One stage in the life cycle is the oocyst which is excreted by members of the cat family (from tigers to domestic cats), especially for a few weeks after infection. Feline infection usually occurs at the kitten age. The oocyst is excreted in the faeces, and may stay alive in soil for up to 18 months.

Another source may be infected meat, but this is becoming less common as deep-freezing the meat and then reheating it kills the organism.

Toxoplasma is transmitted orally.

The infection in adults is asymptomatic in 50% of cases, or may give rise to a non-specific and flu-like illness with lymph gland enlargement, particularly the cervical glands. It is one of the differential diagnoses of glandular fever. Caught in early pregnancy, it may lead to abortion.

Some 80% of women starting a pregnancy are at risk in that they have no antibodies to *Toxoplasma*. Of these, 2 per 1000 pregnancies become infected, and in 40% of cases it is transmitted to the fetus.

Of infected fetuses, 10% go on to show the congenital *Toxoplasma* syndrome, of which the three classical features are:

1. Hydrocephalus.
2. Intracranial calcification.
3. Retinochoroiditis and consequent retinal scarring.

Between 400 and 700 cases occur each year in the UK.

Even if there is no evidence of trouble at birth, later problems may occur. Up to the age of 5 years the syndrome can manifest itself, often as fits. Severe visual impairment has been reported up to age 18. Possibly as many as 80% of infected fetuses show some late manifestations.[4,5]

Recommendations
- Pregnant women should avoid kittens and especially their litter trays.
- Meat should be well-cooked, and vegetables washed.
- Routine serological screening is not recommended.
- Pregnant women should wear gloves if handling possibly contaminated material such as soil and cat litter, and should wash their hands thoroughly after handling raw meat.

Cytomegalovirus

Fifty per cent of people contract cytomegalovirus (CMV), usually in the first few years of life. It causes a non-specific febrile illness with lymphadenopathy, again not unlike infectious mononucleosis.

Ten per 1000 pregnant women contract a primary infection during pregnancy, and in half of cases there will be infection passed to the fetus. Of the infected fetuses, 10% are affected at birth, and a further 10% are affected later. Ten per cent of microcephaly is due

to congenital CMV.[4,5]
The classical picture in cytomegalic inclusion disease is:

1. Blood dyscrasias (thrombocytopenia, anaemia).
2. Low birth weight.
3. Choroidoretinitis.

Recommendation
The virus is transmitted in urine and saliva in the aftermath to an acute infection. It is suggested that pregnant women avoid kissing and cuddling other children as children are the most likely age to have just had an acute episode.

Listeriosis

Listeriosis is rare in pregnancy. Signs and symptoms are non-specific and resemble influenza. In the pregnant woman acute infection may lead to mid-trimester abortion or premature labour. Prompt treatment of suspected cases is advised as early treatment with amoxycillin (or erythromycin in the penicillin-sensitive) may save the pregnancy.

Recommendations

Medical   In a pregnant woman with an unexplained pyrexia of over 48 hours, consider listeriosis. Treatment should be started without waiting for blood culture results.

High-risk foods   Foods often contaminated with *Listeria mono-cytogenes* should be avoided in pregnancy:[6]

1. Soft ripened cheeses, e.g. Brie, Camembert, blue vein.
2. All types of pâté.
3. Cook-chilled meals and ready-to-eat poultry, unless cooked through and piping hot.

Food storage and handling
1. Observe 'use by' and 'best by' dates.
2. Keep the refrigerator cold enough.
3. Separate cooked and raw foods in the refrigerator.
4. Throw away left over reheated food.

Cooking
1. Make sure meat and poultry products are thoroughly cooked

and piping hot.
2. Observe the cooking and standing times recommended when using a microwave oven.
3. Make sure reheated food is hot all the way through.
4. Reheat food once only.

Other precautions *Listeria, Toxoplasma* and *Chlamydia* may be acquired from sheep who are lambing. Pregnant women are advised to avoid contact with lambing sheep.

Where is the best place to be born?

In the past, attending the woman in labour formed a significant part of the work of a GP. Now, however, whereas the majority of GPs offer antenatal and postnatal care to their patients, only a minority offer intrapartum care.

There remains a fierce division of opinion between those who feel that only delivery under consultant care can secure the best likely outcome from the pregnancy, and others who feel that good results can usually be secured with a home or GP unit delivery, with less stress on the mother. Such is the conviction with which these views are held that it is not uncommon for the GP who is not involved in intrapartum care to be asked to justify his or her position by a woman seeking a home confinement.

What are the facts?

Six per cent of pregnancies are delivered by GP in the UK.[7] These include those delivered in GP obstetric units and the 0.5% planned and 0.5% unplanned who deliver at home. In community surveys, 12% of women prefer a home delivery. In the Netherlands 35% of babies are delivered at home.[7]

In 1927 85% of babies were delivered at home.[8] By 1946 this had fallen to 50%.[9]

In 1960, the Association for Improvements in Maternity Services campaigned for facilities to be available so that all babies could be delivered in hospital.

Ninety per cent of GPs offer antenatal and postnatal care, but only 30% offer intrapartum care. The fee for intrapartum care is slightly less than for fitting an intrauterine contraceptive device.[10] The midwife is the senior professional present during 75% of deliveries.

Is home delivery safe?

Data on the relative safety of hospital consultant care, hospital GP care and home delivery safety are skewed by a number of factors.

1. High-risk pregnancies tend to be consultant-booked.
2. Problems during labour usually result in the transfer of the woman to a consultant unit.
3. Not all home deliveries are booked for home delivery.
4. Improvements in women's health generally are probably as important in maternal and fetal well-being as place of birth.[8]

In addition, a number of other trends are occurring which make place of birth statistics hard to interpret:

1. There has been an increase in congenital abnormalities during this century, with the exception of neural tube defects, which are declining.
2. Not all obstetric problems are due to lack of care, for instance only 10% of cerebral palsy is thought to be due to birth care problems.[7]
3. The traditional indices of obstetric care – morbidity and mortality – are now sufficiently rare to make research difficult.
4. There is poor correlation between morbidity and mortality figures and other indices of good obstetric practice. Things may still go wrong even if no mistakes have been made.

Notwithstanding all these confounding factors, the figures for 1979 were as follows. The overall perinatal mortality rate in the UK was 14.6 per 1000. In unbooked pregnancies delivered at home the mortality rate was 196.6 per 1000. For women booked for hospital confinement but who were unable to get to hospital in time the rate was 67.5 per 1000. However, the mortality rate for those babies who had a planned home delivery was only 4.1 per 1000.[7]

The perinatal mortality rates in the Netherlands are comparable with the UK, though many more babies are delivered at home.

Low- and moderate-risk pregnancies are as safe delivering at home as in hospital. High-risk pregnancies are safer delivering in hospital,[8] but some studies have even disputed this.[9]

What do the mothers want?

Women are less happy with maternity services than with any other aspect of health care. As morbidity and mortality statistics cannot be used to justify a particular place of birth, material satisfaction is becoming an important aim of obstetric services. Items shown to influence maternal satisfaction[11] include:

1. The delivery, especially pain experienced, duration of labour, complications.
2. Medical and nursing care received.
3. Information received by the woman and her perceptions of participation in decision-making.
4. Physical aspects of the delivery room.
5. Being treated with respect, and kept informed of progress.
6. The presence of a competent care-giver. Constant attendance during labour has been shown to lead to a significant decrease in perinatal complications and Caesarean sections, and to halve the duration of the labour.[10]

What is the legal position?

Maternity services are separate from general medical services. GPs sign up (on form FP24) each woman separately, and claim a fee from the family health services authority (FHSA) when the care is complete. Care is divided into:

1. Antenatal care from before 16 weeks.
2. Antenatal care from after 16 weeks.
3. Intrapartum care.
4. Postnatal care, plus a separate claim for each postnatal home visit done.

In addition, the GP has a general obligation to render services in an emergency whether or not that particular woman is booked with him or her for pregnancy services.

If you book a woman for intrapartum care, then the requirements in terms of skill are the same as those for a consultant obstetrician. Bolam's Test, which is the requirement only to display the levels of skill of GPs as a class, *does not apply* in this case.[12]

A number of home deliveries are unplanned. The GP who does not undertake intrapartum care may get the impression in the early stages of a pregnancy that a particular woman is not happy with a hospital confinement and intends to delay letting anyone know she is in labour until such time as a home delivery is inevitable. It is important that good records are kept about what you have recommended and what services you have undertaken to provide.

Organization and training problems

Getting involved in intrapartum care either at home or in a GP unit requires a 24-hour commitment. To do the job properly, you should at least be available for the labour, the delivery, and for repairing any episiotomy. You can't rely on the deputizing service or disinterested partners.

Seventy per cent of vocational trainees get obstetric experience,[8] but this is almost entirely in hospital units dealing with abnormal deliveries. It is therefore not particularly suprising that new principals are no more keen than other GPs to undertake deliveries. Different training in GP units or with midwives may alter this attitude.[10]

Each GP is unlikely to have very many deliveries to deal with in a given year. Competence decays faster than confidence, even in the well-motivated. The only practical way to avoid becoming deskilled is to take on other GPs' home deliveries as well – something easily achieved because of the booking system: just as with contraceptive services, you can book maternity services with any GP, not just the one with whom you are registered.

Government policy

The House of Commons Select Committee on Health in October 1992 commissioned a report from the Expert Maternity Group. They reported in August 1993 in a document called *Changing Childbirth*.[13] The main emphasis of this was to promote more community maternity care, and improve information and freedom of choice for pregnant women.

A section called 'Woman-centred care' highlights three areas:

1. It is important that the woman is involved in choices about her care, and that enough information is available to her to make those decisions well-informed.
2. There should be sensitivity to the needs of the local population and community.
3. It is important to secure value for money.

An appendix cites 24 objectives by which progress can be assessed. There is heavy emphasis on maternal choice, flexibility of – especially – midwife services, extra training needs and a trend towards more home deliveries.

The prenatal detection of Down's syndrome

Screening for Down's syndrome

It is estimated that 70% of district health authorities by 1993 had a screening programme for Down's syndrome in place.[14]

By the measurement of chemical markers in maternal blood it is possible to identify a cohort of women who are more likely to be carrying a Down's fetus. The cohort identified are then offered amniocentesis to confirm or refute the diagnosis. It is not justifiable to offer amniocentesis in all pregnancies, because in 0.3–1% of cases the procedure induces an abortion.[15] The alternative of chorionic villus sampling induces abortion in 2–4% of cases.[15]

Previously, amniocentesis was offered only on the basis of maternal age for pregnant women over 35 years old. This only had a sensitivity of 30%, and 7% of pregnant women would be offered amniocentesis.[16]

The biochemical markers in most widespread use are:

1. Unconjugated oestriol.
2. α-Fetoprotein.
3. Chorionic gonadotrophin.

The triple test using maternal age plus the above markers will detect 5% of pregnancies, in which 60% of cases of Down's syndrome will be detected.[17] A refinement of this test, reported in 1993, which uses age, α-fetoprotein and free β human chorionic gonadotrophin, has a 70% sensitivity and a 5% false-positive rate.[18]

It is estimated that it costs £38 000 in 1992 prices to detect one Down's fetus using the currently available screening tests.[17]

Are there any problems with screening?

1. Any screening procedure has to be backed up by counselling, both for the procedure, and for the positive result.
2. The only 'cure' which can be offered is termination of the pregnancy, which some women will decline. Eight per cent of women in the UK are opposed to any form of antenatal diagnostic testing.[14]
3. Amniocentesis carries a small risk of inducing an abortion.
4. Some women over 35 who would have been offered

amniocentesis under the old system will be found to be at low risk, and so will not be offered a test.

5. There is ample evidence that, whatever else a screening programme may do, it certainly generates anxiety among those screened.[19]

The structure of antenatal care

How often do women have to be seen?

Antenatal care was devised in the 1920s as an extension of infant welfare clinics. It was actively promoted by Dame Janet Campbell, who also laid down the regime of clinic visits which has appeared in the textbooks ever since. There is no correlation between the number of clinic visits and the outcome of the pregnancy: in Switzerland the average is five visits; in the Netherlands it is 14.[20]

By tradition, visits are at 12 weeks for booking, then a monthly visit till 28 weeks, fortnightly to 36 weeks, and then weekly till delivery. Originally all routine antenatal care was performed by midwives, with a doctor only being called in if there were problems or if something unexpected happened.

By identifying the tasks of antenatal care, it is possible to rationalize the frequency of clinic visits without losing any clinical usefulness. This would be cost-effective and reduce inconvenience for the patient:[20]

12 Weeks: History and examination. Pregnancy advice.
16 Weeks: α-Fetoprotein and scan.
22 Weeks: Fundal height, baseline weight.
30 Weeks: Assess fetal growth, pre-eclampsia check.
36 Weeks: Assess fetal growth, check presentation.
40 Weeks: Assess need for induction.

In addition, in the primiparous it is suggested that blood pressure, urinalysis and a discussion of delivery and feeding be done at 26, 34, 38 and 41 weeks.

Weighing

In underweight women, poor weight gain in pregnancy is associated with an increased risk of a small-for-dates baby, and a good weight gain ameliorates this.[21] However, this is not true for normal or overweight women.[22] In some centres women are no longer routinely weighed at each antenatal attendance.

Ultrasound scan

The vast majority of pregnant women in the UK are scanned at around 16 weeks. Some reports are appearing about possible fetal changes, e.g. a diminution of left-handed babies in the scanned. Some women also wish a minimum of artificial monitoring of their pregnancies. There is no demonstrable difference in outcome between pregnancies that have and have not had a scan.

An ultrasound scan does, however, seem to be a more accurate way of estimating gestational age than to do this by memory of the date of the last menses.[23] This is important for the woman making plans for the delivery. It is also important so that good use can be made of screening procedures such as the triple test where timing of the blood samples is important.

Glycosuria

Sixty-five per cent of women have glycosuria at some stage of pregnancy. Chemical diabetes is found in only 10% of women who have repeated glycosuria. A blood glucose 1 hour after a glucose load has greater prognostic significance.[21]

Proteinuria

Checking urine for protein is important. In the absence of raised blood pressure, however, the most likely cause of a protein show is a contaminated dipstick.[21]

Abdominal girth

Using a tape measure to assess maternal girth is only 15–30% sensitive in detecting fetal weights below the 10th centile.[21]

Postnatal vaginal examination

Doing a routine vaginal examination at the postnatal examination rarely detects anything untoward in the absence of other symptoms. It can be safely restricted to those women with an indication to have it performed.[24]

References

1. Department of Health. Vitamin A and Pregnancy. PL/CMO(90)11. 1990
2. Department of Health. Folic Acid and Neural Tube Defects: Guidelines on Prevention. PL/CMO(92)18. 1992
3. Gilbert GL. Chickenpox during pregnancy. *Br Med J* 1993; **306**: 1079
4. Best JM and Banatvala JE. Congenital virus infections. *Br Med J* 1990; **300**: 1151–2
5. Ho-Yen DO and Joss AWL. *Toxoplasma* and cytomegalovirus infection during pregnancy. *Maternal Child Health* 1988; **13**: 225–7
6. Department of Health. *While you are Pregnant – Safe Eating and How to Avoid Infection from Food and Animals.* London: HMSO. 1991
7. Young G and Drife J. Therapeutic dilemmas: home birth. *The Practitioner* 1992; **236**: 672–4
8. Jewell D and Smith L. Is there a future for general practitioner obstetrics? *RCGP Members' Reference Book* 1990; 229–32
9. Campbell R, MacFarlane A and Cavenagh S. Choice and chance in low risk maternity care. *Br Med J* 1991; **303**: 1487–8
10. Young GL. General practice and the future of obstetric care. *Br J Gen Pract* 1991; 226–7
11. Smith LFP. Quality, continuity and maternity care. *RCGP Members' Reference Book* 1992; 239–41
12. Day AT. So you want a home confinement? *Maternal Child Health* 1993; 217–18
13. Expert Maternity Group for the Department of Health. *Changing Childbirth.* London: HMSO. 1993
14. Connor M. Biochemical screening for Down's syndrome. *Br Med J* 1993; **306**: 1705
15. Chamberlain G. Detection and management of congenital abnormalities. *Br Med J* 1991; **302**: 949–50
16. Donnai D and Andrews T. Screening for Down's syndrome. *Br Med J* 1988; **297**: 876
17. Wald NJ, Kennard A, Densem JW *et al.* Antenatal maternal serum screening for Down's syndrome: results of a demonstration project. *Br Med J* 1992; **305**: 391–4
18. Spencer K and Carpenter P. Prospective study of prenatal screening for Down's syndrome with free beta human chorionic gonadotrophin. *Br Med J* 1993; **307**: 764–9
19. Statham H and Green J. Serum screening for Down's syndrome: some women's experiences. *Br Med J* 1993; **307**: 174–6
20. Chamberlain G. Normal antenatal management. *Br Med J* 1991; **302**: 7749
21. Steer P. Rituals in antenatal care – do we need them? *Br Med J* 1993; **307**: 697
22. Dimperio DL, Frentzen BH and Cruz AC. Routine weighing during antenatal visits. *Br Med J* 1992; **304**: 460
23. Rowlands S and Royston P. Estimated date of delivery from last menstrual period and ultrasound scan: which is more accurate? *Br J Gen Pract* 1993; **43**: 322–5
24. Noble T. The routine 6-week postnatal examination. *Br Med J* 1993; **307**: 698

12

Loss and bereavement

Aims

The trainee should:

- Be able to identify the stages of a bereavement reaction.
- Be aware of the different possible reactions to a loss.
- Be able to plan a programme of bereavement management.
- Be able to detect if an abnormal reaction is occurring and respond appropriately.

What causes a loss reaction?

When humans are subject to a loss which affects a number of different aspects of their life, a typical reaction results. The circumstance most extensively studied is when there has been a death of a close friend or family member. However, similar reactions occur when a terminal diagnosis has been made, when a part of the body has been amputated or when a job has been lost. Of particular relevance to children is their reaction when their parents divorce.

How common is death?

The death rate in the UK is about 12 per 1000 people per year. A GP with a list of 2000 patients will have 25 deaths among his or her patients each year. Of these, 15 will be over 70 years and 2 will be under 45 years old. At any one time a GP will have up to 2 terminally ill patients. Sixty per cent of people die in hospital.

The chance of being bereaved of a spouse rises with age:

- At age 45–59, 2% of men and 8% of women are bereaved of a spouse.

- At over 75 years this rises to 30% of men and 64% of women.[1]

The population who have had a husband or wife die is thus about 4 million. The average GP will have 135 patients on his or her list who have lost a husband or wife through death.

Why is bereavement important?

The bereaved population will come to the GP's attention in a number of ways:

- *Death.* Being bereaved carries a mortality risk. This is greatest in the first 6 months for widowers and in the second year for widows. Men and the younger bereaved are at greater risk.[1] There is no particular illness which causes these excess deaths, but coronary heart disease and alcohol abuse are well-represented. Suicide is also more common in the first year after a bereavement. In years past, infectious diseases were particularly prevalent.
- *Morbidity.* In the process of a consultation for another matter, it may become clear that a recent death or an abnormal grief reaction has a bearing on the presenting problem.
- *Bureaucracy.* Every death has to be certified by a registered medical practitioner. The terms used on the death certificate may be confusing and need explaining to the bereaved family.
- *Continuity.* The GP will often have built up a relationship over many years with the deceased and family. It is appropriate to continue this care at what is often a distressing time.
- *Efficacy.* There is some evidence that the involvement of a GP or other carer in a counselling role after a bereavement reduces the chance of morbidity in the bereaved.[1]

What are the stages of a loss reaction?

People faced with a loss all go through similar stages of the reaction. The severity and length of each stage will vary, but all can nearly always be identified. The reaction may take over a year to complete, and a duration of up to 2 years is not unusual. The meaning of a loss can only be defined by the person undergoing it.[2] No one can tell you how to grieve.

Shock and denial

This can last for a few hours or up to a week. The reality of the death has not sunk in, as though the patient needs time to catch up with reality. Normal functioning is suspended, so the patient may need help with purposeful thinking and action. The patient may deny or try and bargain away reality. This time is characterized by free-floating anxiety and sleeplessness.

Searching and yearning

This tends to begin about the time of the funeral, and may last for a month or so. The funeral is a particularly important ritual which finally confirms the death so that it can no longer be wished away or denied. Being able to see and touch the body can be an important aspect of this stage. If this contact is denied, either because of circumstances or because a misguided well-wisher forbids it, then this can block the bereavement process.

There may be overactivity of a searching nature. Cupboards may be cleared out obsessively, as though the deceased is being looked for.

Anger and guilt may be apparent. The bereaved is trying to blame someone for the loss. If these feelings are self-directed, then guilt results. It is also not uncommon for anger to be directed at the GP or other doctors involved in the terminal illness. The GP should maintain a professional detachment in these circumstances, but if the anger is too great then that particular GP may have to withdraw from his or her role.

Another feature of this stage is the need repeatedly to go over the events leading up to the death, often in meticulous detail. This can happen particularly when the bereaved has not been present at the death.[3] Allowing the patient repeatedly to review the death is therapeutic, the only response required being to reinforce the fact that neither the bereaved nor anybody else is to blame for the death.

Depression and disorientation

When the funeral is over and the family have returned to their own homes, the real 'work' of bereavement begins. The consequences of the death begin to be realized, leading to waves of acute distress. The distress may be so severe that bizarre behaviour arises, leading the bereaved to think he or she is going mad. There may be a strong sense of the deceased's presence, so that the bereaved may feel that he or she has heard the deceased's voice or more uncommonly 'seen' the deceased, usually in a familiar setting. After years of marriage, couples can predict with some accuracy what their partner is going to do or say in particular circumstances. These memories are so strong that they creep into reality.

Depression is a normal and healthy reaction to bereavement.

Reorganization

The reality of the new world without the deceased is now apparent, and adjustments begin to be made to cope. This stage is the longest and can persist for up to 2 years. Even after this time the deceased is not forgotten, but his or her absence is being tolerated.

Waves of distress may persist, especially when provoked by a memory or an event. During the first year it is always possible to think back to what happened this time last year. Family occasions, birthdays, Christmas and anniversaries are poignant times. Meeting people who are unaware the death has occurred causes distress to both parties.

The resumption of normal social activities, or the first time the bereaved enjoys him- or herself or laughs can trigger guilt feelings again.

What determines the strength of the loss reaction?

The severity of the loss reaction depends on the closeness and quality of the relationship with the deceased. This has been separated into:[4]

- *Strength of attachment*. The closer the relationship, the more severe the reaction.
- *Security of attachment*. This reflects the degree of trust the bereaved had in the relationship.
- *Reliance*. The degree to which the lost person fulfilled particular roles and functions for the bereaved.
- *Involvement*. The degree to which the life space of the lost person and bereaved was shared.
- *Warning*. A sudden and unexpected death will tend to cause a more acute reaction than one which has been anticipated. With an expected death some of the grieving work will already have been done after the fatal diagnosis is made.[5]

How can an abnormal loss reaction be detected?

Up to 30% of those who are bereaved may develop maladaptive

grief.[6] Even with a normal reaction, there may be evidence of significant distress in up to a quarter at 2 years.[5]

In the Harvard Bereavement Study of young widows,[7] it was found that some features were more likely in cases of maladaptive grief:

- Sudden unexpected bereavement. There is difficulty accepting the loss, with distress and strong grief feelings. Longer-term anxiety, depression and social withdrawal are features. At 13 months only 9% had a 'good' outcome, compared with 56% of those who were forewarned of the death.
- Ambivalent relationship with the deceased. The initial distress is less, but the guilt and sense of searching more severe and prolonged (up to 4 years). Thirty per cent have a good result at 13 months compared with 60% of the 'low conflict' group.
- Intense yearning. When all aspects of the couple's life are intertwined, every event is a reminder of the loss. In addition, some skills of daily living such as cooking may need to be learned. A sense of yearning and loneliness persists.

Maladaptive grief can usually be detected because there is failure to progress to the next stage of the bereavement reaction or, put another way, the bereaved has got stuck in one stage. Persisting anger may be a problem, and this can be made worse if an inquest has been needed or if a complaint has been registered about a doctor involved in the care of the deceased. In either of these events there will be a significant delay in all the facts surrounding the death being clarified. The adversarial nature of the current GP complaint procedure means that there is unlikely to be any discussion of the circumstances of the death between the doctor involved and the relatives if a complaint is pending. This can only impede the bereavement process.

Prolonged pining or searching, morbid preoccupation with death, a history of psychiatric illness or persisting guilt all predict a poor outcome. The suggestion that the grief has not resolved often comes from a carer.

Some people never fully work through their grief reactions, and though in many respects they are functioning normally there are none the less signs of distress. Grief may be described with freshness even though the death was years before. Minor triggers provoke intense grief reactions. Themes of loss keep appearing in discussion. The bereaved is unwilling to move the deceased's possessions in an attempt to deny the loss. Physical symptoms like those of the deceased may develop. Radical lifestyle changes may be made.

There may be depressive symptoms or attempts at self-harm.

What can help the bereaved?

Bereavement is a natural and normal process and there is no 'cure' for it. Professional and voluntary carers may supplement the patient's own social support network. A good network of supportive relationships helps the bereavement process proceed in an orderly manner. Short-term counselling can be highly effective in securing a normal bereavement.[5]

The best environment is one in which the bereaved can express their feelings freely and still be accepted. Confidants who have undergone a bereavement reaction themselves are particularly helpful.

In general, carers, either professional or lay, should:

- Be available.
- Listen rather than talk.
- Reinforce the normality of what is happening.
- Accept that there will inevitably be displays of anger, guilt and distress.
- Counsel against major life changes, e.g. moving house in the bereaved period.

Can bereavement be hindered?

Many people find the distress of others distressing. It is very English to show a stiff upper lip and not give way to displays of emotion. Both these factors tend to make carers say and do things which are probably unhelpful to the bereaved.

Unhelpful attitudes identified by the bereaved include;[5]

- Offers of advice.
- Attempts to encourage recovery.
- Forced cheerfulness.
- Identification with feelings such as 'I know how you feel'.

Is medication useful?

In the early days of a bereavement distress may be overwhelming, and sleep impossible. It is often appropriate to prescribe a small quantity of anxiolytic such as diazepam 5 mg three times a day to help the patient over the first day or so. Lack of sleep may be an extra worry in that some people feel that this may lead to illness. Once reassured on this point, night sedation is often declined. Tablets will not cure bereavement, and by reducing awareness may actually impede the bereavement process. Most patients will accept this, and it is not uncommon for only a few doses of the medication to be taken. Confronting the distress head-on is hard work at the time, but probably means that the adjustment to the new reality of life without the deceased progresses more rapidly.

Some patients will welcome their distress and bear it willingly as their way of indicating how much they cared for the deceased, and how much pain they are prepared to endure as a result. It is as though if enough work is put in, then the death will be cancelled, and if not, then it's not for lack of trying.

The routine use of antidepressants does not help the bereaved. It may be apparent, however, as the weeks and months pass that the normal depression is deepening and persisting. In this case the same diagnostic parameters should be applied as when dealing with any depressive illness, so that the severity of the depression and the existence of biological features such as sleep disturbance, low energy and altered appetite will predict whether medication is likely to work. If antidepressants are used, then dosage should be as for other depressive illness, for example tricyclic antidepressants 75–150 mg a day.

How can the GP help?

Breaking bad news

The GP may be involved in telling the family that a death has occurred or is likely to occur. It is important to break the news in such a way that the message is conveyed without causing unnecessary distress:[8]

- Make protected time available.
- Deliver information slowly to prevent denial. Pause between pieces of information.
- Be honest without being brutally honest, and do not make promises you are unable to fulfil.
- Try and assess immediate reaction and answer initial questions at the time bad news is first discussed. Answers may be modified by patient reactions. For some, full details will be discussed, while

for others there may be complete denial.
• Explore the patient's concerns and make time to deal with them.
  It may be necessary to reflect questions to identify real feelings.

At death

Attend promptly – this is not a medical emergency, but it is a social
one. Little can be achieved in terms of counselling, but practical
issues such as undertakers, death certificates, registration of the
death should be addressed. Sometimes physical contact helps.
Medication may be appropriate.

In the few weeks after a death, the bereaved will be deluged with
requests for information. Pension and insurance companies will
often need proof of death. There may be immediate financial
concerns. Further information can be obtained from the under-
taker, from the local social services department or from the
Department of Social Security booklet *What to do after a Death*.[9]

At a housekeeping level, the date of the death can be entered
into the bereaved's medical records. This can be useful in future
contacts. Any hospital departments should be notified. There is
little more distressing for the bereaved and embarrassing for the GP
than the receipt of an outpatient appointment for the deceased.

After the funeral

• The family have gone home and the house is empty. Around 2
  weeks the bereaved will experience lots of guilt feelings and
  searching. They will want to go through the details of the death.
• Explain anything on the death certificate which is not understood.
• Discuss the events leading to the death if the patient wishes.
• Describe the normal bereavement reaction and its normality.
  Feeling angry and depressed is normal, as is seeing and hearing
  the deceased.
• Assess what support is available. This may be family, friends,
  clergy, voluntary groups.

Around 4 months

• The initial grief is often starting to resolve. Assess progress and
  look for problems. It may not be necessary to do anything if
  there is good support.
• Assess the need for further contact. At this stage it should be
  clear whether or not the bereavement is likely to be normal. If

there seem to be problems, then further contacts may be organized either at home or surgery.

• If pathology is developing, then:

Increase the frequency of contact with the patient. Occasionally a clinical depression may occur, which should be managed like other depressions using tricyclics if necessary.

Refer on to either to a professional or lay colleague.

Advise contact with a self-help group such as CRUSE (126 Sheen Road, Richmond, Surrey TW9 1UR. Bereavement lines: Counselling 0181 332 7227; Information 0181 940 4818). Many churches provide support for the bereaved.

What are the special problems of children?

The response of children to loss is in many ways similar to that of adults, but modified by their own perceptions.[4] Deaths of first-degree relatives are rare, but loss through divorce causes reactions just as severe as death, and by some measures (e.g. incidence of enuresis) causes more problems.[2] Similar reactions can be seen after the loss of a pet, or even after moving house.

The loss of a parent in childhood is associated with an increased chance of psychiatric disorders, particularly depression, in adult life.

• Aged under 6 months, the baby has no concept that people continue to exist when they can't be seen, and so there is no separation anxiety. Under 2 years, children have no idea of the permanence of death.
• From 2 to 7, children see the world only from their own viewpoint, and may feel responsible that the loss has occurred.
• From 7 to 12, there is acceptance that death is not their fault.
• Over 12, abstract thinking is such that hypothetical situations can be speculated on.

Typically, the following stages are gone through:

1. Protest – anger, crying, looking for the parent.
2. Despair – depression, hope of reunion lost.
3. Emotional detachment – recovery is apparent, but the capacity to form deep attachments is damaged.

A pathological reaction in a bereaved child is suspected if there is prolonged depression, scholastic failure, social isolation of more than 3 months, inability to play, antisocial or aggressive behaviour, drug or alcohol abuse, delinquency, sexual 'acting out', prolonged somatic symptoms or thoughts of suicide or dying.[2]

References

1. McAvoy BR. Death after bereavement. *Br Med J* 1986; **239**: 835
2. Furnivall J and Wilson P. Coping with loss in childhood. *Med Monitor* 1991; **15**: 51–4
3. Freeman R. Supporting the grieving patient. *Med Monitor* 1991; **4**: 33–4
4. Furnivall J and Wilson P. Coping with loss in childhood. *Med Monitor* 1991; **4**: 56–62
5. Preston J. The consequences of bereavement. *Practitioner* 1989; **233**: 137–9
6. Yates DW, Ellison G and McGuiness S. Care of the suddenly bereaved. *Br Med J* 1990; **301**: 29–31
7. Parkes CM and Weiss RS. *Recovery from Bereavement*. New York: Basic Books. 1993
8. McLaughlan CAJ. Handling distressed relatives and breaking bad news. *Br Med J* 1990; **301**: 1145–9
9. Department of Social Security. *What to do after a Death*. DSS leaflet No. D49. London: HMSO

13

How to get a job as a general practitioner

Aims

The trainee should:

- Be able to make a list of mandatory and desirable features to look for in a practice.
- Be able to prepare an appropriate curriculum vitae (CV).
- Know the mechanisms available to find a practice vacancy.
- Be able to prepare for an interview.

What are the important statistics?

In 1985, the number of trainees completing vocational training was 30% higher than the number of GP posts which became vacant.[1] Demand for vocational training has declined by 80% since the new contract was introduced in 1990, so that now there are an average of 2.5 applicants for each vocational training scheme (VTS) post compared with 12 in 1988.[2] This has not yet filtered through to the numbers emerging as certificated GPs, which is remaining constant at around 2100 a year.

Jobs become available in three ways: a vacancy in an established group practice, a single-handed vacancy or setting up from scratch in an 'open' area. According to the Medical Practices Committee, in 1987 there were 1867 inclusions on to the medical list, of which 1700 were doctors joining existing group practices. There were an average of 43 applicants per single-handed post, of which 130 were filled in the year. Very few new practices were started.[3]

A survey in 1985 of a group of recent ex-trainees[4] showed that it takes an average of 20 weeks and 19 applications to get a job. Between 2 and 14 months after finishing a VTS, 52% were full-time principals, 11% were part-time, 6% were working as locums, 5% were waiting to take up a post, and 5% were working as a salaried partner or an assistant. This leaves 21% unaccounted for, some of whom will have gone overseas, and some who will have left general practice either temporarily or permanently.

From the same survey, 33% were offered a job without even making an application, nearly always in the area where they had been a trainee. Another 25% found their job via ads in the *British Medical Journal*.

What do trainees want?

A survey of 140 delegates at the seventh national GP trainee conference in June 1993[5] found that only 24% intended to go straight into work as a GP principal. Thirty per cent wanted to do locum work, and 11% wanted to go back and work in hospital at least for a time. Another 30% expressed a desire to work abroad.

Eleven per cent wanted to leave medicine temporarily, and 1.5% wanted to leave permanently, with a further 3.5% wanting to go into an associated medical field. This will be of particular concern to government, as each GP costs about £180 000 to train.[2]

Looking at preferred types of practice, 50% of trainees would consider a suburban post, 40% a rural location, but only 8.5% were looking for a job in the inner city. Thirty-five per cent of trainees are looking for job-sharing posts.

A further survey of trainees in the North West Thames region[6] found that 28% would consider working in inner London. Twelve per cent said they would be prepared for single-handed practice, and 28% would work in a practice of two.

What are the implications for GP recruitment?

General practice is thought by many medical students to be limited in scope and increasingly overburdened with bureaucracy, though the financial rewards in the short term are seen as better than staying in hospital work.[2]

The anticipated rise in the population of 4.3% between now and 2011 will require a further 1400 GPs if present list sizes are sustained.

These factors should mean that it is now a seller's market for jobs in general practice. In reality, the move to capitation fees and an attempt to maintain income have encouraged many practices to increase their list size by not filling practice vacancies, or by taking on new doctors as assistants rather than as partners.

It is hard to predict how many GPs will leave practice and so create vacancies. There is some anecdotal evidence that more GPs are planning to retire early, and the option to retire at 50 will doubtless encourage this. It is not inevitable, however, that earlier retirement will lead to more jobs on offer.

What is your ideal practice like?

Most trainees have a pretty good idea of the sort of practice they want to end up working in. This is often very similar to their training practice – the clone effect. However, only 25% of practices are training practices, and they are selected to conform to particular regulations. These regulations may or may not be consistent with your idea of a good general practice.

While it is important to have a good idea at the outset of the sort of practice you are after, it is impossible to find one which will fit in with every requirement. It is useful to draw up a list of desirable characteristics, and then establish which of them you would and would not be prepared to compromise on, forming a mandatory and desirable list.

While compromise is inevitable, it is important to exercise some care in choosing a practice, even if this means not being able to go straight into a new job when vocational training is complete. There are plenty of ways to spend your time until the right practice vacancy comes along. You will be spending more time at work than you will with your spouse, which should indicate the level of care needed in choosing a suitable job.

Factors to be taken into account when choosing a practice are:[7]

- *Practice area.* The work and social role of the GP can be very different in a rural area when compared with urban practice. Dispersed rural practice may sound ideal, but there is less back-up and more travelling, which may make the workload very high from time to time. A practice with a base in a 'nice' area may have patients in the less salubrious parts of town, or may have little pockets within the area where problems tend to be focused.
- *Number of partners.* Small partnerships can be more friendly, and there is usually less inertia when practice changes are needed. There is usually more continuity of patient care. On the other hand, interpersonal squabbles become magnified.
- *Number of patients.* Dividing the list size by the number of doctors gives a bare idea of workload. A sight of a map of the practice boundaries will show how dispersed the patients are, giving an indication of problems with home visits.

- *What are the partners like?* The age range, sex and special interests of the other partners will give an idea of what the practice is short of in terms of GP skills. The age structure will show whether any more partners are due to leave. An old-style autocratic senior-partner-run practice may be (but is not always) intolerant of change and development.
- *Practice premises.* Practice-owned buildings have to be bought into, so money has to be found. If the practice dispenses, this will add an average of £80 000 to the buying-in costs.[8]
- *Income.* The list size and achievement of targets will give a broad indication of likely income. Income will also depend on starting share, time to parity and buying-in arrangements. The time to insist on seeing the books is not, however, until after the interviews.
- *Workload.* The way the on-call is organized can make a difference to workload and income. Deputizing services can ease the workload burden considerably, but are expensive. Inequitable work-sharing causes problems and resentment. There may be differences between partners in the number of surgeries or amount of on-call being done, often justified on the pretext that 'we had to do it when we were junior partners'.
- *Practice organization.* The presence of a practice manager will tell you a lot about the practice's attitude towards organization and efficiency. The manager very rapidly becomes pivotal in how the practice works, and the character of the manager is thus of importance. A practice agreement should exist and be in good order. Many practices use the introduction of a new partner as an opportunity to update the agreement. The existence of clinics and ancillary staff should be checked, as well as any problems with staff members. Does the overall practice philosophy accord with your own?
- *Local hospitals.* The availability of a range of secondary care facilities and investigative procedures can make a big difference to the pattern of work. The presence of adequate postgraduate education facilities is desirable.
- *Local amenities.* Will you and your family enjoy living in or about the practice area? What are the schools, cultural and leisure facilities like?

How can I find out about job vacancies?

It is usually easier to find out about job vacancies which arise in the area you are already working in. You will have contacts and have established a reputation. You will also be seen to be committed to the area and so less likely to want to move on. Sources of information are:

• Ads in the *British Medical Journal* or one of the free medical newspapers.
• Word of mouth from colleagues or course organizers.
• The Family Health Services Authority (FHSA) will know of posts falling vacant. Some will offer to circulate your CV for you.
• The Local Medical Committee (LMC) will often be prepared to help.
• Advertisements in the local postgraduate centre.

How can I get short-listed?

Having chosen a practice you wish to apply to, the next task is to get short-listed. It helps if you already know the practice and they know you. Make sure that any other information they have about you works to your advantage. The game's afoot to leave a good impression.

Before the application, find out as much as you can about the practice and the area. This helps you make a choice, and also informs your application. Talking to people in the local pubs and shops can be illuminating.

Contact the practice and ask to visit. If you have visited, ring up later to thank them and express your continuing interest.

If a locum becomes available in a target practice, try and do it. You will get a much better idea of how the practice works, and it is also a good chance to get yourself known by the partners and, perhaps as importantly, by the rest of the practice staff.

What should be in the curriculum vitae?

This is often the first information the practice will have about you. It will arrive along with a variable number of others, and time spent on presentation will make it stand out from the rest.

Try and make it well-spaced-out, and legibly printed. Access to a word processor is extremely useful as lots of good-quality copies can be made, and it is also possible to alter the text for each application. Use lots of headings. Be concise.

Include details of education back to secondary school, including any prizes. More detail is needed for your medical education, but try and stick to aspects relevant to general practice.

Your work career so far should get the most attention and detail. Do not try to cover any gaps as they are very easy to spot. If you spent a few months ill, or climbing in the Himalayas, then say so. It might even help – a consumer's view of the NHS can be quite instructive.

The front page of your CV is most accessible, and should include nearly all the relevant information, even if this is expanded later in the text. Suitable items for the front page are:[9]

Personal details

Name in full, address, date of birth, marital status, spouse's career, children, nationality.

Work details

Confirmation that you hold a driving licence. General Medical Council registration number. Defence society membership number.

Work background

Medical school details. Preregistration jobs. Postregistration jobs. Postgraduate qualifications. Training practice experience.

Names of referees

In the ensuing text, topics can be expanded. Remember, however, that more than three pages of even the brightest prose is unlikely to be fully read.

Feelings are mixed about whether or not to include a photograph with the CV. Some people feel that something of their character can be communicated in a photograph better than in text. Some candidates will wish to emphasize a particular aspect of their character and so will include a photo which also shows the spouse and children and occasionally the family pet. In general, jokes do not work, so remember what impact your photo is likely to have and consider whether this is the sort of impact you want to make.

If a photograph is used, it should be an original print, and a reasonably accurate likeness. Photocopies of photographs and the little passport-sized items which you get from the machine in Woolworths always make you look like the trainee from hell. Have due regard to the aesthetic sensitivities of your putative partners.

What should go in the covering letter?

The covering letter is your main way of impressing the partners. It should be written by hand, but legibly. Try and think what you would want to know if you wanted a new partner. Competence is often assumed from the training and any further qualifications, so this is only part of the issue.

Connections with the area go down well. If you know the area already, and have other reasons to stay, you are more likely to stick with the job. The commonest time for a partnership to break down is in the early years. Frequent changes in partnership take up a lot of time and are stressful.

Your research of the area may have given you some extra insights into the problems and possibilities the practice may have. Include these in your letter. It might also be worth making the odd suggestion about the future of the practice, but err on the side of caution as the other partners will always know more about the problems than you do.

Tell them why you want to go into general practice, and why you want to join them. All GPs think their way is best, and have invested a lot of effort in getting things the way they are. Stroke a few egos.

Include something about non-medical interests. The zealot is regarded with suspicion, but then so is the laggard. Don't exaggerate, as sooner or later you will come across a real expert who will easily call your bluff.

Show them you have at least read the ad. Try and address any issues specifically raised (e.g. 'eligible for obstetric list') and indicate how you would deal with them.

Practices all have to be managed. Any interests or special experience you may have in administrative areas should be covered either in the CV or letter.

What do partnerships look for?

In a study in 1993,[10] 110 GPs in the North West region were asked what qualities they would look for in a new partner:

- 75% preferred an applicant under 35 years old, and 57% preferred a married applicant. Children were thought an advantage by 45%.
- 35% wanted an innovative partner, and 20% wanted an extrovert, while only 8% wanted an introvert.
- 65% expected some postgraduate qualifications, of which

MRCGP and DRCOG were favourites. However, 20% felt that 'too many' qualifications would be a disadvantage.

- 30% preferred a local applicant, and 55% would appoint their own trainee.
- Obstetrics/gynaecology, paediatrics and general medicine jobs were seen as desirable postgraduate experience by over 80% of appointing GPs.
- 65% of practices put ads in the press 6 months or more before the vacancy arose, so the aspirant partner should plan early.

How should you conduct yourself at the interview?

Once short-listed you will be required to attend one or a number of interview situations. You are being assessed during them all, even the 'trial by sherry'. Be on time and look the part.

Try and be yourself as far as the circumstances will allow. Joining a practice is making a contract, not winning a prize. If you create a false image which you cannot or do not intend to sustain, then they will get a distorted image of you and you of them. This will inevitably lead to longer-term strains in the relationship.

A self-opinionated approach is usually disliked – they are looking for someone who will fit in with them. Philosophical and religious views are usually strongly held. If you or the practice have particularly strong beliefs in areas which may affect the day-to-day work of the practice, then it is as well to get them out into the open at an early stage. Disagreement on such things can lead to a lot of future problems, and it's no good hoping you can convert them all.

Listen to the questions, and try to answer them.

Most GPs haven't the faintest idea how to interview, and may well be as nervous as you are. Those who are organized will have looked carefully at what they think the practice needs in a new partner, and will be looking for someone to fulfil those needs. It may be possible from your research to predict what characteristics are being looked for and respond accordingly.

You are interviewing them as much as they are interviewing you. You will need to know certain things about the practice, and a checklist doesn't go amiss. Many of the questions may well have been answered in informal discussion, but you will need some information on all of the following:[11]

How do things work?

- How many GPs and staff are there?

- How is the workload shared out?
- What is the list size? Are any changes expected?
- How is out-of-hours cover organized – deputizing, rota, etc.?
- What attached staff are there?
- Are the practice annual reports available?
- What about fundholding? If not, are there any plans? Locality commissioning?
- Are any specialist services offered?
- What is the health promotion band achieved?
- Is there scope for outside appointments?
- Does the practice dispense?
- Is the practice computerized? Are there any links with the FHSA?
- Are there any special allowances, e.g. deprivation?
- What sort of medical records are used? Can they be viewed?

Money

- How many years is it to parity?
- What are the profit-sharing arrangements?
- Are there any special clauses in the agreement, e.g. building up one's own list?
- Are all earnings pooled – outside jobs, seniority, Post Graduate Education Allowance (PGEA)?
- Is there provision for maternity/paternity leave?
- Can you see the practice accounts?
- Who owns the premises?
- What are the buying-in arrangements? How are valuations made?

Philosophy

- How are relations with local providers?
- Is the FHSA regarded as helpful or obstructive?
- Are higher targets being met, e.g. child health surveillance?
- Are team meetings held?
- Is it a training practice?
- What is the attitude towards staff training?
- Are there any plans for a nurse practitioner?
- Are there any prescribing policies? Is there a practice formulary?
- What is the attitude towards private patients?
- How are practice decisions made?
- What is the attitude towards external advice, e.g. management consultants?
- What are the audit arrangements?
- Is there any provision for sabbaticals and study leave?
- Is the practice keen to innovate?

Lifestyle

- What are property costs like?
- What are local schools like?
- How many partners have children?
- Are there any sporting facilities available?
- Are there any leisure facilities available?

Should you be concerned about money?

The short answer is yes. You are entering a small business venture from the more reliable environment of salaried employment. Everyone else will be acutely concerned with making a living, and in a partnership you have responsibilities to them as well as yourself.

Working out your earnings

When you have been offered a post, it is important to look at the practice accounts before accepting. They should be shown to your own accountant for an assessment. If the accounts are not forthcoming or are not for the latest available year, then either mismanagement or a deception may be assumed. There may be undisclosed debts which need to be serviced. The post is unacceptable.

Profit share and time to parity should be laid down in the partnership agreement, as should details of any capital required. If it is shown separately, it will be possible to work out how the practice compares with the average with respect to getting the various claims in. Income per patient for a number of items of service is published monthly in *Medeconomics*.

It is typical for a new partner to join at half a parity share. This may be negotiable, for instance in the case of older doctors with family commitments, especially if they are moving practice and thus suffering a cut in income. Working out how your entry in the partnership will affect the profits is a bit more complex:[12]

- Be clear what you are getting a share of. Many practices pool all earnings, but in others PGEA, seniority, outside jobs and training grants are kept by the earner.
- Outside jobs and seniority may well be lost with the retiring partner. This will affect profits.
- Some expenses may alter when you join, for instance the need to employ locums.

- Notional and cost rent reimbursements may appear in the accounts. If you are not buying-in you will not get a share of these, but neither will you bear the loan finance costs.
- The accounts will include details of the partners' personal expenses. You will inherit part of these but it takes a few years to build them up to a decent level, and this will affect your tax liability.

The future earning power of the practice is more difficult to predict. A falling list size spells trouble. Overheads tend to stay fixed as you cannot unbuild premises, and sacking staff is not fun.

Tax

Until 1996, the tax liability of a partnership is the responsibility of the whole partnership. If you are joining a partnership, you will almost certainly be asked to sign an election of continuation of partnership. This means you are liable to pay tax from day one rather than a year in arrears, as would happen if you were setting up alone as a self-employed worker.

After 1996 (with a transition period from 1994), tax liability becomes the responsibility of the individual and tax is worked out based on a current year earnings estimation. This means that you are not liable for tax payments after you retire, which is exactly the same as if the partnership had continued to require continuation of partnership agreements from incoming partners.

Capital

All practices have capital assets, even if it's only fixtures, fittings, drugs, etc. These have to be bought. In addition, all practices need a certain amount of working capital. These are not usually huge sums (unless its a dispensing practice) and can be covered painlessly.

Since 1965, there have been considerable incentives for GPs to invest in premises under the Cost Rent Scheme. This is a highly advantageous way of borrowing money, and most GPs do it. However, it does mean that the capital assets of the practice are much higher, and this puts an additional financial burden on the incoming partner.

In general, you will be paying off the outgoing partner, and some sort of loan will usually have to be taken out. This will often be done in stages reflecting your current profit share, which is the method most consistent with partnership law. Alternatively, you may not be liable until you reach parity.

Another option is that you are not required to purchase any of the partnership assets. This is unusual since the outgoing partner will need to be paid off, and the partnership is likely to work better if all have an interest in its financial health.

The costs of buying into the partnership have to be borne at a time when domestic expenditure is likely to be high. You may be moving house, a more reliable or a second car may need to be bought, your spouse may be changing jobs. While you are liable for a part of a partnership debt, however, you are also entitled to your share of notional or cost rent reimbursement.

Details of the buying-in arrangements should be contained in the partnership agreement.

How important is a partnership agreement?

The partnership agreement contains all the details of the agreement you have with your partners. Without one it is impossible to work out whether you are going to be treated fairly by the other partners. This runs the risk that you will suffer abuse, and also means that there is huge potential for disagreement within the practice.

It is important that the agreement is written down. Do not join a practice which has not got a partnership agreement.

Model partnership agreements can be obtained from the British Medical Association. Before signing an agreement, show it to your solicitor. An agreement should include:[13]

- Constitution of the partnership.
- Commencement date.
- Practice premises and equipment.
- Rental or purchase details.
- Residential restrictions.
- Annual, study and sabbatical leave.
- Other absences: maternity, compassionate.
- Division of income: private and NHS.
- Profit-sharing ratios.
- Profits relative to list size.
- Liabilities for debts, taxes, gifts.
- Accounting procedures.
- Banking and accounting details.
- Access to practice finances.
- Other medical commitments or businesses.
- Retirement and expulsion.
- Grounds for termination or dissolution.

What are the common pitfalls?

Horror stories are always circulating about how new partners have been misled and abused when joining a practice. Few of these methods of abuse are new, and indeed in some cases merely reflect what was standard practice years ago. Senior partners may be genuinely unaware that their behaviour is unfair, and will be glad to learn that normal practice has changed. In other cases the seniors may be trying to compensate themselves for their own abuse when they joined the practice.

- Check how parity is defined. Outside jobs, seniority payments and PGEA may be excluded from the share-out and kept by the individual doctor. Selling goodwill in a medical practice is illegal. If it takes more than 3 years to get to parity, the partnership may be open to a charge of selling goodwill.[14] Some practices pay partners on the basis of their personal list size, which clearly disadvantages the new entrant.
- Ensure that there is parity in workload. The new partner should not be responsible for more than his or her fair share of surgeries or on-call duties. If a deputizing service is used, it should be available to all partners.
- Make sure the buying-in arrangements are fair. A way of valuing the practice assets should appear in the partnership agreement. It is important that the current market value should be used. For equipment this can be worked out by dividing the purchase cost by the likely life of the equipment, much as is done when claiming depreciation against tax. For premises there may be a conflict of interest where property prices have fallen significantly, especially where notional rent reimbursement has fallen behind the loan repayments.
- Look out for hidden costs. It was not unusual in past years for the incoming partner to be asked to buy the retiring partner's house, often at an inflated figure. Expensive loans or unexpected financial obligations on the practice should be spotted when you show the practice accounts to your accountant.
- Be suspicious of previous bad practice. If a partner is leaving for reasons other than retirement, try and find out why. Check the FHSA records for details of previous partners who have left. It is lucrative for a practice to have a succession of partners who never get to parity. This can be done by forcing partners out of the practice, or by refusing to honour parity agreements.

What are the special problems of women?

Women currently constitute 26% of GP principals, and 54% of all GPs under 30 years old.[15] Most work full-time, but they are more likely than men to work part-time or job share, and to be assistants rather than unrestricted principals.

Sexual harassment can range from sexist or patronizing behaviour, through suggestive remarks to unwelcome physical contact. Awards made by industrial tribunals in such cases are relatively small but likely to increase.

Violence is not a problem restricted to women, but they may be seen as easier prey. From 1 April 1994 it has been possible to remove a violent patient from the list with immediate effect. The Offences Against the Person Act can be used in cases of actual assault, and the Public Order Act 1986 makes it illegal to use 'threatening, abusive or insulting words or behaviour that is likely to result in harm or distress'.

Sexual discrimination is illegal in partnerships of two or more. As well as overt discrimination, breach of the legislation can be assumed if, for instance, there is no provision for time off for antenatal care, or the provision for maternity leave is any less favourable than the provisions for illness absence. Questions about child care arrangements and family plans are in strict terms illegal. It is understandable, however, that your future partners would want to know about any factors which might have an impact on workload. When attending an interview it is as well, so long as there are no objections, to volunteer the information.

Part-time work

Part-time work is commoner among women. Under the GP contract, full-time means over 26 hours a week for 42 weeks a year. Three-quarters is 19 hours, and half is 13 hours. Under partnership law this should entitle you by law to a minimum of one-third, one-quarter and one-fifth respectively of the profit share of the highest paid partner.

What constitutes a part-time commitment in terms of surgeries and visits and clinics done, on-call and administrative duties varies enormously from practice to practice. In general you will tend to end up doing slightly more than half the work for half the pay. At any rate, it is difficult to do the work of a GP on a strictly part-time basis as there will always be problems with which only you can deal, and they may occur at any time.

What if I don't get a job straight away?

Your ideal job is unlikely to be available right away. It is important to have a good look around and see what is available before making a decision you will have to live with for the next 30 years.

- You will have direct experience of at most two different practices. They are training practices and so not typical.
- Retirement vacancies become available when people retire, not just to fit in with the end of the local VTS.

There are a number of ways to fill any work gaps profitably.

1. Take some time off. You will probably need a break anyway, and this may be the last chance you have to take prolonged leave.
2. Do locum work – there is plenty available at the moment. This not only plugs the gap, but it also gives you the chance to work in other practices. At the present British Medical Association recommended locum rates it should be possible to get an income approaching what you would expect when joining a partnership.
3. Do some more hospital work. Some trainees welcome the chance to gain experience in other specialist areas.

References

1. Law J. Fill the job gap fruitfully. *Medeconomics* February, 1988; **9**: 85–90
2. Laws C. I don't want to be a GP. *Medeconomics* March, 1994; **15**: 73–81
3. Farish S. Plan ahead to find the right job. *Medeconomics* September, 1988; **9**: 97
4. North MA. Evaluation of the experience of trainees seeking employment after completion of their vocational training. *J Coll Gen Pract* 1985; **35**: 29–33
5. Thomson R. Are you one of the new breed of GPs? *Medeconomics* December, 1993; **14**: 62–3
6. Beardow R, Cheung K & Styles WMcN. Factors influencing the career choices of general practitioner trainees in North West Thames Regional Health Authority. *Br J Gen Pract* 1993; **43**: 449–52
7. Vincent P. Choosing a practice. *Update* 1993; **47**: 52–5
8. Thomson R. Do your homework before you buy in. *Medeconomics* January, 1994; **15**: 57–8
9. Roberts J (ed). Curriculum vitae. *Pulse 'in Practice'* 1989; **49**: 77–82
10. Khunti K. Applying for a partnership. *Update* 1993; **47**: 304–7
11. Sunson S. Interview checklist. *Medeconomics* July, 1993; **14**: 49
12. Slavin S. Assess the earning power of your new practice. *Medeconomics* February, 1993; 96
13. Slayson M. Becoming a practice principal. *The Practitioner* 1994; **238**: 270–3
14. Sean J. What to watch out for when choosing your practice. *Monitor Weekly* 1994; **7**: 57–9
15. Women in general practice. *GP Newspaper* April 1 1994; 76–9

Managing your money in the early practice years

Aims

The trainee should:

- Be able to keep adequate records to inform relations with the Inland Revenue.
- Be able to take a medium- and longer-term view of personal financial planning.
- Understand the impact of short- and long-term illness on financial security, and be able to plan appropriately.

Some background

General practitioners in the UK are self-employed. There are a number of proposals in the pipeline to give GPs the option of salaried work, but this is unlikely to be widespread for the foreseeable future.

GPs as a group have protected their self-employed status with much vigour. The argument is that it keeps the GP independent of the state and so able to deliver personalized care to patients unfettered by outside interference. There are also considerable tax advantages enjoyed by the self-employed, but securing these takes a bit of planning.

The Doctors' and Dentists' Review Body (or just Review Body) is charged with advising the prime minister on the remuneration of doctors and dentists working in the NHS. It is composed of 8 people with backgrounds in accountancy and management in health-related and other industry.[1] There are no doctors or dentists. Each year, after taking evidence from the interested parties, it produces a report which the prime minister receives in January with a view to implementation in the following April.

The Review Body has the broad support of the professions and government as it avoids direct negotiations and disputes between the parties involved and so prevents the consideration of any action such as a strike or a work-to-rule which would interfere with patient care. In order for the system to work properly, the Review Body has to be truly independent, and its findings have to be agreed with.

In 1993, for the first time, the Review Body refused to produce a report as the government had already announced that there was to be a pay ceiling in the whole public sector.

In its report the Review Body recommends a level of gross and net income for GPs. This means that not only is the take-home pay of GPs calculated, but there is also a figure given for expenses. The figures for the year from April 1994 are £64 031 gross and £41 830 net.[2] This takes account of average expenses of £22 501 and a 'clawback' (i.e. an unintentional overpayment from previous years) of £353.

This figure of take-home pay of nearly £42 000 will mask a wide variety between GPs.

- Some practices will be more efficient than others in claiming all their items of service entitlements.
- A number of GPs only do the minimum 26 hours at the practice. They are deemed to be full-time by the Family Health Services Authority (FHSA), but will not be drawing a full parity share of practice profits. This also distorts figures about the average GP list size.
- Non-NHS income is not included. Practices with significant private work can boost their income considerably.

All this means that the average full-time GP will earn more than the £42 000, and the only way you can work out how much you might get in a particular practice is to look at the accounts and try and guess what the future might bring.

When you join a partnership, you are eligible for the benefits of the profits of the partnership. You and your partners are also collectively and severally liable for its debts, including tax liability, but this will change in 1996. If a partner does not pay a debt, then you are liable for it. You are inextricably financially bound to your partners. Any lapse or error can be expensive and may cause a partnership dispute.

What can I claim against tax?

One of the benefits of being self-employed (schedule D tax) is that work expenses are eligible for relief if they are 'wholly and exclusively' incurred by the job. For the salaried employee on pay as you earn (PAYE; schedule E tax), expenses are only allowed if they are 'wholly, exclusively and necessarily' incurred. That one word, necessarily, can make a huge difference, and is very much subject to how the Inland Revenue defines it.

Tax relief on work expenses is allowed at the top rate paid, which for most GPs will be 40%.

Expenses may quite properly be claimed against tax for:

- Motoring. This includes petrol, repairs and servicing, road fund licence, insurance, breakdown organization membership, car rental costs, parking costs and any other expenditure arising because of motoring (but not fines imposed through parking or motoring offences). Relief is also available on loans taken out to buy vehicles, and on the depreciation of vehicles of 25% per year subject to a maximum of £3000 (1993 prices).[3] When you sell a car, however, the actual amount you sell it for is taken account of for tax purposes. It is usual to make claims for two cars in case of breakdown.

- Staff and clerical. This will include salaries of employed reception and nursing staff, as well as recruiting, training and advertising costs.

  It is also legitimate to pay your spouse for practice work, such as telephone answering on-call and clerical assistance. This is most beneficial if the spouse is not otherwise working, but it may still be worthwhile if the spouse is paying a lower rate of tax than the GP.

- Telephone charges, both practice and domestic.

- Subscriptions, journals, postage and stationery.

- Drugs and requisites.

- Household costs. When the GP's private dwelling is used for consultations from time to time, it is not hard to convince the Revenue of the legitimacy of a claim for household expenses.[4] In other cases, a small amount may be claimed for other practice work done at home, or for equipment used for work purposes but kept at home. If dangerous drugs are stored, it is permissible to claim for the installation and servicing costs of a burglar alarm.

- Bank charges. Accountancy and legal costs. Clothes cleaning. It is assumed that a GP will wish to maintain a clean and tidy appearance.

- Pension plans and superannuation.

- Study courses and other expenses.

- Repairs and renewals. You cannot claim relief on new equipment unless it is a replacement for existing equipment. Don't invest in the most expensive stethoscope and ophthalmoscope when you are a trainee, but wait till you are on schedule D and then replace them with something decent.

- Locum insurance. It is wise to insure yourself against locum costs for cover against prolonged ill health. The premiums are allowable against tax. Other policies to insure income if you are permanently unable to work are not allowable.
- Any other expense for the purpose of the practice.

Professional indemnity insurance is a significant professional expense. Even if it is paid through the practice, it should appear as a personal expense in your own accounts.

What tax records should you keep?

Some practice expenses such as rent, rates, staff costs and locum charges are best monitored by the practice administrative team. Most GPs will not be involved directly in this expenditure. Expenses generated in this way are shared round the partnership.

Other expenses may be paid for by the practice and so appear in the main practice accounts. Practices vary in this regard, so in some cases defence society membership and motoring expenses may be paid by the practice, while in others they fall to the individual doctor.

The third category of expenses is those which are paid partly by the practice and partly by the doctor. This might include stationery costs.

Other expenses are entirely the province of the individual doctor, and will include subscriptions.

For the convenience of the practice and the Inland Revenue, a number of allowances may be agreed in advance. This saves the GP having to produce proof of the expenditure and saves the Revenue having to investigate. Practices which have been subjected to an Inland Revenue investigation will attest to the time and effort it takes.

Any agreed amounts have to be broadly reasonable and not substantially out of step with other practices. Sometimes an agreed amount is supplemented by a claimed amount. An example might be a practice-agreed amount for stationery, with a further claim being made by the individual GP for proven extra expenditure.

In other cases it will be possible to claim for a proportion of the expenditure on a particular item. Typical of this type of agreement is the situation where a proportion of motoring costs are allowed so that you do not have to keep a car or cars just for practice use.

If the practice centrally is not keeping a record of expenditure which it may be possible to claim against tax, *then you should do so yourself*. Records kept should be:

- In a book to form a permanent record.
- Recorded at least monthly. Supported where possible by vouchers (receipts).

Motoring expenses are often the most difficult to keep a track of. It is useful to keep a credit card to be used only for motoring expenses. The monthly accounts are adequate proof that the expenditure has been incurred.

What about a pension?

Just having started a new job, and struggling with a below-parity income, perhaps a new mortgage and car loan, a young family and a spouse unable to work because of domestic responsibilities or relocation, it is perhaps an odd time to be considering pensions. None the less it is important to give the subject a little thought for two reasons:

- This is the cheapest time to buy 'added years'.
- You may be approached with a proposal to leave the NHS pension scheme (NHSPS) to join a commercial pension scheme.

The NHSPS costs you 6% of your superannuable income, which after tax relief is about 3% of your NHS income. In addition the FHSA pays a further 4%. This money gathers to form a notional pension fund which pays out on retirement.

The benefits of the NHSPS will vary with individual circumstances. Booklet SDP gives a guide to its major details, and further advice can be obtained from either the pensions officer at the FHSA, or direct from:

NHS Pension Scheme
Hesketh House
200–220 Broadway
FLEETWOOD
Lancashire FY7 8LG
Tel: 01253 774632 or 01253 774635.

In broad terms the NHSPS pays an annual pension on retirement, plus a lump sum of 3 years' pension. Maximum benefits are payable after 40 years' service. The pension is index-linked to the retail price index, and since the scheme is indemnified by the government, it is as secure as you can get.
Other benefits include the following:

- If you die, there is a pension for any surviving spouse and school-age dependants.
- Death gratuity if you die while still in post.
- Partial and total disability benefits.
- The British Medical Association continues to negotiate improvements in the scheme even though you have left practice.

Other pension schemes

There are no independent advisers who are suggesting that GPs withdraw their contributions from the NHSPS. A commercial pension offering the same level of benefits, in particular the index linkage, would be very expensive. In addition, on leaving the NHSPS you forgo the FHSA contribution to your pension fund.

Up to the age of 35 you are allowed to contribute up to 17.5% of income to a pension fund and claim tax relief on all the premiums. This goes up with age, so that over 61, 40% can be paid in.[3]

The A9 concession is only allowed by the Inland Revenue for GPs and dentists. Under this you can opt to forgo all tax relief on NHSPS contributions, and instead claim relief on premiums paid to another scheme. The percentage of income payable is increased, and the income for assessment purposes also includes private earnings. To benefit from the A9 concession you have to want to and be able to pay more into an independent scheme than you pay to the NHSPS. This really only makes sense if you have a lot of spare cash which you want to invest in a tax-efficient way.

Topping-up the pension

Added years
Many GPs will want to retire before they have completed the full 40 years' service which provides a maximum pension. It is now possible for GPs to retire at any age after 50 (except on the grounds of ill health), but the pension you get is correspondingly smaller. This shortfall can be compensated for by buying added years of pension benefit.

You approach the NHSPS and apply to buy the added years. With their agreement, extra contributions to the scheme are subtracted from income before the FHSA pays you. The FHSA makes no contribution to added years agreements. The earlier you start buying added years, the cheaper it is. Exact details of how much it will cost can be obtained through the FHSA pension officer.

Private additional pension
There are other ways of topping-up pension through the private sector, and buying added years is not particularly cheap. Some GPs will find the security of a government scheme more compelling than relying on the ups and downs of the stock market.

If you wish to top-up your pension with a private scheme, this can be done by approaching an insurance company of your choice, by having a financial adviser arrange it for you, or by approaching the Equitable Life Insurance Society with whom the NHSPS has negotiated special terms. Since the commission obtained by brokers for some of these policies can approach half the premiums for the first few years, any scheme which reduces costs is worth looking at.

How can I work out what pension I will get?

In practice this is very difficult. If you apply to the Fleetwood office, they will give you an estimate, but this can only be relied upon in the year or so immediately before retirement. Superannuable income is not the same as actual income for two reasons:

- Private earnings are not included.
- Some parts of income are assumed to be a reimbursement of expenses, and these are not superannuable.

This second factor makes entitlement particularly tricky to work out. A proportion of the total is deemed to be superannuable, and this varies from time to time and between different FHSAs. The current average is that 64.5% of FHSA income is superannuable.[2] Alternatively, the superannuation you pay in a year (figure available from the FHSA quarterly returns or the practice accounts) is 6% of your superannuable earnings.

The contributions which you and the FHSA make are paid into a personal pension fund. The retirement pension is 1.4% of this fund per year. Clearly inflation has meant that money earned years ago is not as valuable now in purchasing terms. This is got round by the use of dynamizing factors. These are set each year, and are figures by which actual money earned in a past year is multiplied to compensate for inflation. The dynamized amount is then added to the pension fund.

How can I work out how much I will need?

This will depend on your plans and priorities, and so no one can tell you. It will probably become a lot clearer as you get older, and this is also the time when you may have some spare money to do something about it. The sort of questions worth asking yourself are:

- Will the house be paid for?
- Will the children be independent?
- By how much will professional expenses fall?
- What will motoring and holiday requirements be?
- Do I intend to have a significant estate to leave?
- Will I want to move house?

Can retirement income be increased in other ways?

In the early years in practice there are many pressures on the income and it is probably not necessary to get too much into debt to build up the pension at this stage. Bear in mind when planning any extra provision that there will almost certainly be extra assets in the form of lump sums available at retirement which can be used to top-up the pension:

- The lump sum from the NHSPS.
- Your share of practice assets.

The cost rent scheme is a highly advantageous way of borrowing money. Practitioners who have used the scheme in the recent past will have an asset realizable on retirement of £100 000 or more, bought essentially with an interest-free loan. This will contribute substantially to pension provision.

What insurance cover should I have?

The NHSPS provides a small amount of life insurance cover, but this is not much in the early years of service. Term life assurance can be taken out reasonably cheaply when you are young and fit. The cover should be enough to pay off your debts and give the family some security. Around £200 000 is suggested, but bear in mind that this will seem a lot less in 20 years' time.

Any loans taken out for substantial purchases (house, surgery) will invariably require some sort of life cover assigned to them. An endowment policy is only a 'with profits' life assurance assigned to a loan, and so provides life cover as well as paying off the loan on maturity.

Dying is relatively easy in insurance terms. Inability to work because of temporary or permanent ill health is more difficult, especially as the cost of living if you are disabled will probably go up.

The partnership agreement should contain details of what happens within the practice if a partner is unable to work because of ill health. It is usual, for instance, for a partnership to agree to provide cover for the first month of any sickness absence. The practice agreement should be read in conjunction with the statement of fees and allowances as, depending on the average partnership list size, time in post of the sick doctor and the duration of absence, the practice may be eligible for locum payments from the FHSA.

If locum payments are available, as a maximum they are paid after a deferment period of 1 month, and thereafter at full rate for 6 months and then half rate for 6 months. It is usual for a practice agreement to require that the absent partner is responsible for meeting any locum costs incurred after the first month. The locum payments are insufficient to meet the British Medical Association recommended rates for a locum, so the amount has to be topped up. Locum payments will only be made if a locum has been employed.

The key times in this scenario are after a month (when a locum is employed), after 6 months (when the locum fee diminishes) and after a year (when the locum fee stops). A number of insurance companies provide locum insurance policies to top-up locum costs where benefits are deferred for the right length of time.

After a year's absence it is not unusual for the practice agreement to stipulate that the partnership dissolves, and your income with it. It is possible to insure against this by taking out permanent ill-health insurance. The cost of premiums varies according to the size of benefit, and none of the ill-health policies will pay out more than 75% of final earnings in benefit. Index-linked benefits are best.

What is the best way to buy my share of the practice capital?

All practices need some working capital, and have some practice assets such as drugs and equipment. The sums involved are much greater if there is property involved. Any outgoing partner will want his or her share of practice assets, and this is normally paid for by the incoming partner.

It is always a good idea to check the buying-in procedure before accepting a partnership. The details should be in the partnership agreement. Raising a large lump sum on relatively low earnings when there are other sizeable expenses can be difficult.

If the capital involved is small, some practices allow the new partner an interest-free loan paid off over 3–5 years. With larger amounts, buying-in may be deferred until parity is reached. The method in closest accord with the legislation governing partnerships is for the incoming partner to be responsible for a share of capital proportional to profit share, so that if you start on a half-parity share of profits, then you are responsible for half a share of the capital of a full-parity partner.

Many young doctors will want to buy their share of the capital assets of the practice as a retirement fund, especially as through the cost rent scheme the purchase can be done at such favourable rates. Many commercial lenders on the other hand are prepared to allow you not to pay off the loan capital, so long as they continue to get their interest. The assets will remain with the partnership after you leave, and the debt will remain a partnership rather than a personal debt. If you wish to pay off the capital, the options available are broadly similar to those available for house purchase, with the difference that tax relief at the highest rate paid is available on the interest for the whole loan.

While you are liable for a full share of the loan, you are also eligible for a full share of any cost rent or notional rent reimbursement from the FHSA. It is not unusual for all the interest to be covered by reimbursments, so that the only outlay for the GP is to pay off the capital. For a healthy GP under 40 years, a low-cost endowment policy over 20 years maturing at £100 000 will cost around £200 a month.

What are my financial priorities on entering general practice?

- Make sure that the Inland Revenue is aware that you wish self-employed tax status.
- Make sure you are on any lists for which you are eligible, e.g. obstetric list, child health surveillance list.
- Have a good close look at the accounts, and show them to your

accountant. This should be done before signing the practice agreement.
- Think what would happen if you died in the near future.
- Think what would happen if you were unable to work through ill health in the near future.
- Make an initial appraisal of your pension provision. Check you are a member of the NHSPS. Consider added years. Other investments in pensions can be left till later, when you might have some spare money.

References

1. One-minute Guide in Practice and Money Matters. *GP Newspaper* October 1993; 62
2. Medeconomics Database. *Medeconomics* Vol 16, no 1, January 1995;
3. *Budget Taxation Guide November 1993*. Chartered Accountants. Sheffield: Barber, Harrison and Platt. 1993

15

Prescribing in general practice

Aims

The trainee should:

- Know how to prescribe effectively and economically.
- Know how to help patients use their medicines to full advantage.
- Be aware of the legal requirements and responsibilities of the prescriber.

Facts and figures

The writing of a prescription is one of the commonest activities of a GP. Around 65% of consultations end with a prescription being issued, and at any one time about 40% of the British population are using a prescribed medication.[1]

Over 420 million prescribed items are dispensed each year from primary care, at a total cost in 1992/3 of £3600m (a rise of 14% on the previous year), or 10% of the total NHS budget.[2] Each GP prescribes on average prescriptions to the value of three times his or her salary.[3]

Rising costs

The amount spent on GP prescribing has remained remarkably constant over the years as a proportion of total NHS expenditure. However, in money terms the costs rose 30-fold between 1961 and 1991, and the number of items issued per GP went up by 50%.[3]

Medical inflation
Medical inflation always runs ahead of general inflation since with new innovations more diseases can be treated. This goes for therapeutic and investigative procedures as well as for medication.

Elderly people
Elderly people use more medicines than younger ones. It has been estimated that people over 75 receive an average of 24 prescribed items per year compared with 12 for the 60–75s, and 5.3 for those aged 16–60.[4] The number of elderly people is increasing, and this will continue to cause prescribed items to rise.

International comparisons

British GPs are frugal prescribers when compared with their overseas colleagues. Using figures from 1989, the consumption of pharmaceuticals per patient per year in the UK was £32. This compares with a highest of £94 for Japan, and a lowest of £24 for Spain. In terms of prescribed items per person, the UK level is 6.5, compared to a lowest of 4.7 for Sweden and a highest of 35 for Japan.[5]

Measuring the prescribing rate

Several factors beside numbers of patients will influence the numbers of prescriptions issued. PACT (see later) uses the idea of the prescribing unit which makes allowance for the reality that some patients need more medications than others. The ASTRO-PU (age, sex and temporary resident originated prescribing unit), has been developed which divides the age bands into nine groups, distinguishes male from female, and also includes a figure for temporary residents.[6] From 1994 this became the basis for the prescribing rates recorded through PACT.

Compliance

Encouraging healthy behaviour in patients is a central role of doctors. In considering the use of medication, a three-way relationship exists between patient, doctor and medicine. The word compliance has authoritarian overtones which implies that if medicines are not used correctly, then it is always the fault of the patient. However, the tolerability of the medicine also has a bearing on the patient's drug-taking accuracy, and it is known that the doctor can employ strategies which make compliance more likely. Despite its limitations, compliance is the only word available.

Partial compliance, that is, when medicines are taken but not as prescribed, is virtually universal.

Non-compliance, where medication is not taken at all, probably has different psychological origins[7] and is much rarer. Here the patient will attend regularly for review, will usually cash in the prescription, and then either throw the tablets away or more normally hoard them.

Primary non-compliance

Anything between 5%[7] and 20%[8] of prescriptions don't get dispensed at all. In a large study from 1993,[9] more women than men were involved, the peak ages being 16–29 for women and 40–49 for men. Some types of medication were overrepresented, with nearly 25% of prescriptions for the oral contraceptive pill not being dispensed. Also, patients who pay prescription charges are twice as likely not to get their prescriptions dispensed.

What else can go wrong?

A number of patients fail to take enough medicine. This may be because of forgetfulness, or because the regime does not fit in with their daily routine. In general, doses of more than two tablets a day are more likely to cause problems. Some patients are quite consistent in their pill-taking and so for instance will not take more than two tablets at a time or more than two doses in a day.

The timing of dosages can cause problems, and drug instructions could be aggravating this. Does 'three times a day' mean three times during the day only, or should it include the night hours?

Many patients will not take medication for long enough. Symptomatic remedies and those such as antibiotics where the patient usually feels better before the course is completed, may well be stopped prematurely. Treatment for chronic disease tends to be taken rather more accurately, as long as the patient is convinced of the value of doing so. The daily routine also tends to alter to accommodate the pill-taking.

A few patients will consistently exceed the prescribed dose. The reasons for this are not known.

Data from one study[8] for β-blockers in angina and hypertension showed that 46% of patients took between 80 and 120% of the prescribed dose, and 20% were fully compliant.

Why won't patients take their medicines?

Health beliefs
Patients tend to take medicines accurately if they perceive it as important for them as individuals to do so. The condition being

treated has to be perceived as serious, or the patient has to feel vulnerable to the consequences of not being treated. This perceived vulnerability is most strongly influenced by anecdotal information from friends or family members. For instance, if a relative had a stroke because of hypertension, then the patient is more likely to comply with his or her own hypotensive treatment.

Supervision
The closer patients are supervised, the more likely they are to take the medicines properly, so that, for instance, 98% compliance may be achieved for inpatient treatment of tuberculosis, but this falls to 50–65% in outpatients.[8]

Proxy supervision, using mechanical devices to dispense the medicines or to monitor when the pills are taken, has been used successfully. Blood or urine drug levels can be assayed. Chemical markers can be put into medication so that compliance can be monitored.

Duration of treatment
The longer the course, the less likely it is to be complied with. However, even short courses can cause problems. In children given a week's course of penicillin, by the third day the drug can be detected in the urine of 46%, and by the sixth day it is down to 31%.[8]

Complexity of drug regime
With more different drugs and increased daily dosage, more doses are likely to be missed. Best compliance is achieved with one or two doses a day – higher than this the compliance falls off.

Patient satisfaction
If the patient's concerns and expectations have not been addressed during the consultation, it's hardly suprising that he or she is less likely to take your proposed treatment seriously. It is estimated that in between 1 and 3% of consultations the presented problem is not the chief problem,[7] and this group of patients are particularly likely to leave dissatisfied.

Information and explanations are valued by patients. Any increased anxiety is offset by increased satisfaction. Time taken to discuss the ailment and the effects and side-effects of treatment is time well-spent. From January 1994, EC Directive 92/27 requires a leaflet to be included in all original packs dispensed, including details of what the drug is, what its indications are, how to take it, what side-effects are possible, the expiry date, and other information necessary before use, for instance, contra-indications, precautions, interactions.[10]

What can the GP do?

- Simplify the drug regime.
- Tailor the regime to the daily routine.
- Involve the patient in monitoring the condition.
- Make sure the patient understands the condition and the treatment.
- Make sure the patient is in agreement with your assessment of the problem and the proposed treatment.
- Hand out appropriate leaflets where available. Around half of patients would like more information about their medicines. Remember that when producing leaflets, the average reading age of the British public is 9 years.[11]

Does compliance really matter?

The people keenest on estimating the effects of non-compliance are the drug companies who want to make sure that their products do not fail to work because they have not been taken as recommended. This is somewhat spurious for the clinician who at the end of the day wants to know if a treatment used on free-living patients will actually bring about the required benefit. If a treatment works but has lots of miserable side-effects, it is not likely to be taken properly. It doesn't really matter if the the drug doesn't work or the patient won't take it – the effect is the same.

Dosages of drugs are worked out at the research stage by reference to animal experiments, and these doses are then used in human trials. Since human and animal physiology is not the same, choosing the final dose is a bit of a lottery, and the manufacturers tend to err on the overdosage side to ensure clinical effectiveness. Frequency of dosage is a little easier to determine from monitoring blood levels.

Overall therefore the dosage regime which is eventually recommended is one which is known to work. On the other hand there may be other ways of using the same drug which are equally effective, but which haven't been subject to trials. Work on antibiotic regimes, for instance, has shown that 3 g doses of amoxycillin are as effective as 7 days of smaller doses in treating urinary tract infection.[12] Most children don't take their penicillin for more than 3 days anyway.

More research work on abbreviated and simplified drug regimes would be clinically and economically very useful.

Regulating new drugs

Each year in the UK around 600 new licences for pharmaceutical products are granted. Of these, about 5–10% are for completely new drugs (new active substance or NAS), and the rest are already established products in new doses, formulations or combinations.[13] Most NASs are variants of existing medications, for instance a different β-blocker or H_2 antagonist. An innovation such as the first β-blocker or H_2 antagonist is very rare. It is economically safer to exploit an existing market.

Each NAS costs the drug industry about £100m to find and develop, and up to 14 years of the current 20-year patent may be used up getting the product licensed and on to the market. Only around 20% of NASs eventually end up making a profit,[13] so it's not surprising on commercial grounds that the majority of 'new drugs' are in fact old drugs in new clothes.

The 1968 Medicines Act provides the legal regulatory framework governing the supply and use of medicines in the UK. This act is based on the recommendations of the Sainsbury Committee which was convened after the thalidomide tragedy.

The Medicines Control Agency (MCA) administers the act. It oversees the manufacture, promotion and distribution of medicines, and can inspect factories in the UK and abroad and check for purity of ingredients.

The Committee on Safety of Medicines (CSM) was set up by the Medicines Commission which advises health ministers on implementation of the Medicines Act. The CSM advises on questions of efficacy, safety and quality of new medicines.

For a drug to be sold in the UK it must hold a product licence granted by the MCA. The licence is granted if the MCA feels the product is effective, safe and can give overall benefit. Its deliberations specifically exclude considerations of comparative efficacy, that is, whether it is better or worse than existing products. The product licence specifies the name, nature, method of manufacture and quality of the medicine. It also stipulates what the drug can be used for, and at what dosage it is approved.

Sufficient evidence has to be produced to convince the MCA that a licence should be issued. After initial research looking at the pharmacology and toxicity of the product in animals (usually dogs and rats), a suitable dose and formulation for human trials is worked out. Human trials fall into four phases:[14]

- *Phase I*: Clinical pharmacology in normal volunteers.

- *Phase II*: Clinical investigation to confirm the efficacy and likely dosage range.
- *Phase III*: Formal therapeutic trials to establish efficacy and safety in 1000–3000 volunteers. At this stage data are submitted to the MCA for a licence.
- *Phase IV*: Postmarketing surveillance. Rare toxic effects need large samples to become apparent. Many thousands of patients will be involved.

How is drug safety monitored?

When a new drug receives a product licence, the manufacturer will have had to convince the MCA of the safety of the product. Rare adverse effects, however, often do not become apparent until the drug has been in general usage for a time, as this is when sufficient numbers of patients will have used the drug for the rare side-effects to emerge. At the stage a licence is granted, there will have been up to 3000 patients taking the drug. Tens of thousands of patients may be exposed before a rare effect becomes apparent.

Postmarketing surveillance

The drug manufacturers conduct their own trials on new products. This is usually done by the company approaching a clinician (GP or hospital doctor) to monitor the effects of their treatment. There are strict guidelines regulating the conduct of and the remuneration for such trials (see later).

Yellow card scheme

This is run by the CSM. Clinicians are invited to fill in a yellow card if they suspect that a drug has caused an adverse reaction. Cards can be found in the *British National Formulary* (*BNF*) and *Monthly Index of Medical Specialities* (*MIMS*) in the NHS prescription pads, in the Association of British Pharmaceutical Industry's (ABPI) data sheet compendium, or obtained direct from the CSM.

New drugs, marked by an inverted black triangle in *BNF*, *MIMS* and the data sheet, are of particular interest, and any adverse effect, however minor, should be notified. For older drugs, interest is focused on severe reactions, even if they are well-recognized as side-effects.

Only a minority of GPs send in yellow card reports, which must reduce the effectiveness of the scheme.

Prescription event monitoring

This is run with government support from the University of Southampton. Drugs in which they are interested (usually new products) are identified from prescriptions. The prescriber is then sent a form to fill in with questions on the indications for the drug, whether it worked, why it was stopped, and whether there were any events during or after its use. Typical events include obvious reactions to the drug, and also accidents and surgery seemingly unconnected with the medication.

Using this information reports on efficacy and safety are produced and circulated.

How are drug prices agreed?

The drug industry in the UK is highly successful in commercial terms. Exports in 1988 were £1730m, and there was a positive trade balance of £890m. Some 87 000 people were employed direct and a further 250 000 relied on the industry for their jobs.

A total of £720m was invested in research and development (R&D) in 1987, representing 16% of all R&D money spent by UK industry, even though the drug industry accounts for only 2% of UK industrial sales.[15] Much of this money goes to academic research establishments – though most drug innovation derives from the industry itself, in some instances the products of research are 'bought' from universities.

After a number of instances of profiteering, the Pharmaceutical Price Regulation Scheme (PPRS) was set up to agree target profits with the drug companies. The current basis of agreements is that the companies should not make more than between 17 and 21% profit each year on the capital employed.[16] The PPRS has as part of its remit an obligation to support the industry and the national economy, and this is also taken into account when the company profits are agreed. The final agreement is confidential, and though profit guidelines are published, the actual profits agreed with companies can lie outside these figures.

Drug company profits

Total drug sales in the UK in 1992 were £4250m. Of this, £3400m was sales to the NHS, and the rest sales through pharmacies. PPRS applies only to branded products, so 14% or £470m of sales were excluded from its influence.[16]

On average the industry spends 8% of its sales revenue on promotion.[16] As 80% of this is on GPs,[17] this represents over £7000 worth of promotion for each GP each year. The Department of Health can sanction companies which overspend their promotion budget. The use of the money in terms of gifts and hospitality is governed by a voluntary agreement between the ABPI and the government. Details of this agreement are to be found in the data sheet compendium which the ABPI publishes roughly annually.

Postmarketing surveillance

The involvement of GPs in postmarketing (phase IV) surveillance has caused some concern. The industry is encouraged to do such surveys, and primary care is an obvious place to do them. The GPs involved might reasonably expect to be paid for their work.

However, in some cases the reimbursements were out of proportion to the work involved and might be considered as inducements to prescribe the particular drug.

In other cases the study survey designs were so poor that they were unlikely to yield useful information. Once a GP begins a medication which works, it is very difficult to change again to an older and cheaper product even though it may be just as good. Hence the company has acquired a market for its product under a thinly veiled pretence at research.

Guidelines on the involvement of doctors in phase IV studies have been agreed by the ABPI, British Medical Association, CSM and the Royal College of General Practitioners. These can also be found in the data sheet compendium.[18]

Generic prescribing

Once a new drug is out of patent, anyone can make it. The manufacturer who patents and licenses the drug bears all the development expense, and may have only a few years left of the patent in which to recoup those costs. The maker of the generic can thus make and sell the drug more cheaply.

In the quarter ending November 1993, 49% of drugs were prescribed using generic names.[19] The dispensing pharmacist has some discretion with a generic prescription whether to dispense a generic or a branded equivalent. Roughly two-thirds of generic prescriptions are dispensed using generic drugs.[20] Occasionally a company will market a branded product at a lower cost than the generic equivalent – the so-called branded generic.

All generic medications are subject to the same tests of safety and efficacy as their branded counterparts, and need a product licence. In the UK around 80% of generics are made by eight companies, seven of which are subsidiaries of larger firms making branded products.[21]

In some cases it is specifically recommended that generics should not be used. Where there is a narrow therapeutic window, as with antiepileptics and theophyllines, even small changes in bioavailability may lead to loss of therapeutic control. Also, licences are not issued to generic slow-release preparations.[21]

Reasons to prescribe generically

- In most cases the generic product is cheaper and just as effective as the branded product.
- The generic name indicates more about the pharmacological group the drug is in than does the contrived brand name.
- All medical students and trainees are taught using generic names.

Reasons to prescribe branded products

- The tablets will always be the same size, shape, colour and taste. This gives patient confidence and maximizes the placebo effect.
- Generic names are harder to remember and spell, with increased scope for error.
- The excipients in generic products (the material that is not drug) will vary, leading to different bioavailability.
- The proliferation of generic prescribing undermines the profitability of new innovation. The UK drug industry is important for the economy of the country.

Parallel imported medicines[22]

The dispensing pharmacist will want to buy drugs at the lowest price so that profits are maximized. In some cases drugs can be obtained overseas at lower prices, and in some instances those same drugs have been made in the UK, then exported. When the UK joined the Common Market, the Treaty of Rome dictated that there must be free passage of all goods, including drugs, between member states.

The MCA will issue a licence called a Product Licence Parallel Import (PLPI) to a drug which is essentially similar to one which

already holds a product licence in the UK. There are strict regulations to make sure that labelling and any leaflet are in English.
The pharmacist will retain any savings made by parallel importing. Patients may be slightly perplexed to receive their normal medication with a label partly in Greek.

How to prescribe economically

The four criteria for rational prescribing are well-established. The drug being prescribed should be:[23]

- Necessary.
- Safe.
- Effective.
- Economic.

Necessary

Many of the conditions seen in general practice are self-limiting. Prescribing antibiotics for all sore throats when the majority will be viral wastes resources, runs unnecessary risk of side-effects from the medication, reinforces a particular health-seeking behaviour, and undermines the confidence of the patient to look after his or her own health needs. If patients start presenting all their symptoms to the doctor, and not just the 10% which is currently estimated, then the service would be rapidly overwhelmed.

Safe

All medicines available in the UK have their safety certified by the issue of their product licence. This does not rule out, however, patients with special risk factors such as renal failure or pregnancy who may be particularly susceptible to adverse drug reactions. It also does not allow for problems arising from drug interactions.

Effective

The efficacy of a medicine is also ensured by the licensing body who base their judgement on the evidence presented to them when the licence is sought. Postmarketing surveillance and other trials may subsequently show that the drug does not do what it is claimed to do. Good examples would be drugs used for intermittent claudication which have no proven benefit, or those such as appetite suppressants which are no longer recommended.[24]

Economic

New drugs
GPs in the UK are less likely to prescribe newer drugs than their overseas conterparts, despite the expenditure on promotion. In 1987, 9.3% by value of prescribed drugs in the UK had been launched in the previous 5 years, the lowest in a range up to 29.3% in Italy.[5] New drugs are nearly always more expensive than older ones.

Real benefits
In many cases more expensive treatments offer true advantages over older ones, and patients should not be deprived of these. Care must be taken when interpreting the evidence. Improved side-effect profiles may not be translated into clinical importance: for instance, altered lipid levels are only important if they lead to disease. Rare side-effects may not be apparent until many years of clinical use. It is unlikely that any new drugs will be recommended as safe during pregnancy because of the problems of having a cohort of patients to test them on.

Overall health costs
Some medicines may be more expensive in the short term but save more costly operations or other treatments in future. Some cytotoxics have so many side-effects that they can only be given in hospital, whereas the more expensive equivalent can be used at home. An injection into a shoulder joint may be more economical in the long run than a course of physiotherapy.[5]

Rules for economic prescribing[24]

- Prescribe only when the benefits of the medicine are likely to outweigh the risks.
- Only prescribe a drug if the patient intends to take it.
- Prescribe only remedies of proven efficacy.
- Where drugs are identical in terms of safety and efficacy, then prescribe the cheapest version.
- Prescribe for the shortest period that is clinically indicated.
- Prescribe using generic names.
- Monitor prescribing. This is equally important for repeat

prescribing, as up to 65% of all items prescribed are done without the patient being seen.[23]

Prescribing analysis and cost (PACT)

PACT was devised by the Prescription Pricing Authority in 1988. Every 3 months, data from prescriptions are collated and sent to GPs. At its most detailed it gives a 99% accurate individual picture of a GP's prescribing habits.[25]

1. Level 1 is a four-page report sent unsolicited to every GP. Comparisons between the practice and local and national averages are made as regards number of items prescribed, cost per item and overall cost. Inside is more detail in six therapeutic areas where national costs are highest, these at present being: cardiovascular, gastrointestinal, musculoskeletal, respiratory, infections and others. On the back are details of the individual GP's prescribing in terms of generics prescribed and items per patient.

   Prescribing rates are not based on raw patient numbers, but on the ASTRO-PU (see earlier). This takes account of the fact that different types of patient will normally require different numbers of medications.
2. Level 2 gives more detailed data, specifically in high-cost areas. You receive level 2 data automatically if the practice prescribing costs are 25% above the Family Health Services Authority (FHSA) average, or if the cost in any therapeutic group is 75% higher than average.
3. Level 3 is only obtainable on request. It is a full breakdown of all prescriptions by BNF grouping, with the costs of each. It is a bulky document and takes quite a long time even to read. However, it gives invaluable information about the details of a practice's prescribing, and is an ideal place to start if you are producing a practice formulary.

What about a practice formulary?

Changes in prescribing behaviour can be achieved by a constant review of performance. Each GP has a personal formulary which is developed by habit, tradition (personal and the patients he or she inherits), anecdote and sometimes informed choice. About 10% of GP practices have their own written formulary,[26] and over half of

GPs are in favour of having one.[27] In addition, around 50% of hospital pharmacies have their own formulary.

Formularies are not new. In 1862 the General Medical Council produced the first *British Pharmacopoeia* (*BP*). After the 1911 National Insurance Act each GP was given 6 shillings per patient plus another shilling for medicines, so that prescribing economy was paramount. The Liverpool formulary of 1913 contained 31 preparations, all in Latin.

The first *BNF* was brought out in 1949. It now contains about 4000 preparations, and is updated every 6 months, with each revision needing about 4000 changes. It is not just a list of drugs, but also contains details of their use and recommendations.

How do you write a formulary?

- Find out what your prescribing habits are through PACT level 3 data and/or by looking at your repeat prescribing data.
- Look at one of the published general practice formularies.
- Look at the local hospital formulary, if available. Care should be exercised on prices, however, as drugs can be sold more cheaply to hospital pharmacies than to the community.

Making progress

No formulary should seek to cover all clinical situations, especially the complex ones where a number of drugs are being used. Tests on the Lothian Formulary showed that it could be used in 75% of clinical situations.[26] Any formulary seeking to do more than this will tend to be very complicated (thus undermining one of the main reasons for having it) and may well restrict clinical freedom.

The educational process of constructing a formulary is at least as important as the finished product. A group of drugs, or a *BNF* section, can be selected for review. Advice can be obtained from the literature and from community and hospital pharmacists. The aim should be to agree on a 'best buy' in each category, with a few further recommendations if the first choice is not to be used for some reason. The same process can then be repeated in other categories of drug.

The final formulary should not be prescriptive, but if it is 'owned' and agreed by the practice it is more likely to be followed. On the other hand, some favourite prescribing habits may be challenged by the formulary. It is often more tactful to change prescribing habits by criticizing a formulary developed elsewhere rather than challenge the established habits of a senior partner.

Writing a formulary is time-consuming. The Northern Ireland Formulary took 30 hours of discussion to develop, and in another case a formulary designed to cover only half of prescribing took 8 hours of meetings to devise.

Reasons to have a practice formulary

• To rationalize prescribing.
• To coordinate hospital and GP prescribing.
• To save money. This effect may not be significant. A move to generics will help, but underuse of some drugs (for instance, inhaled steroids in asthma) may be identified. Also greater emphasis on economy may lead to non-drug but more expensive treatments being used.
• To educate the people who have devised it. Including other professionals in the compilation also promotes team-building.
• To form the basis for discussing management policies within the practice.

Reasons not to have a formulary

• It restricts clinical freedom.
• It promotes generic prescribing.
• It delays the use of newer drugs.

Some legal considerations when prescribing

Product liability

Up until 1988 patients who wished to make a claim that they had been damaged by a drug had to prove that someone had acted negligently. From the enactment of the Consumer Protection Act 1987, from 1 March 1988 the idea of strict liability was introduced. Under this the claimant only has to prove that the drug has caused damage, not that anyone has been negligent. The responsible person is the manufacturer or the importer if the drug is made outside the European Community.

If the manufacturer/importer cannot be identified, then responsibility is passed down the dispensing line and may eventually fall on the prescriber. To avoid litigation it is therefore important to make sure that a line of responsibility for each drug dispensed can be established. Dispensing GPs will have considerable problems.

For non-dispensing GPs most drugs can be traced back at least to the dispenser, and this then becomes the dispenser's problem. In two circumstances extra care has to be taken:

1. Drugs dispensed 'from the bag' in emergency.
2. Items altered before administration, for instance bending a hypodermic needle invalidates the manufacturer's guarantee.[28]

Guidance from the British Medical Association[29] urges members to:

- Adhere strictly to labelling requirements when dispensing drugs. This includes the patient's name, details of the supplier, date dispensed, and the words 'keep out of reach of children' or similar.
- Record the details of drugs dispensed in the patient's notes. It must be possible to identify the manufacturer from this, so generic names are less useful.
- Keep accurate records of invoices for at least 11 years.

Unlicensed drugs or unlicensed indications

A product licence, among other things, specifies what the drug can be used for. In many cases the drug is effective for other indications, but getting a new indication licensed is expensive and the manufacturer may not consider it worth the money for the possible extra sales.

If an unlicensed drug is used or a drug is used for other than a licensed indication, then the prescriber is responsible for any problems which arise. Avoiding this responsibility may deprive patients of helpful treatments. For instance, tricyclics are not licensed for use in pain control, but in some situations are very effective.

If a prescription for an unlicensed drug or an unlicensed indication is being considered:[30]

- The doctor has a duty of care to the standard consistent with the practice of a responsible body of peers.
- The doctor should be fully aware of the implications of his or her actions and be prepared to defend him- or herself.
- The patient should be made aware of the circumstances, and informed consent obtained.

Informed consent

Doctors have a clear professional obligation and a legal duty to explain, in terms which the patient can understand, the nature and purpose, the significant adverse effects, the possible complications and the appropriate alternatives of any treatment they recommend.[28] When there is a high risk of side-effects, either through severity or frequency, then the fact that the patient has been warned of the risks should be noted. An example would be drowsiness from benzodiazepines in a lorry driver.

Clinical responsibility

The doctor with clinical responsibility for the condition being treated should issue prescriptions for that treatment.[31] Particular problems arise at the GP–hospital interface where for reasons of patient convenience or economy a GP is invited to prescribe medicines initiated by a hospital colleague.

- A GP who is unhappy taking clinical responsibility for a particular medicine should not prescribe it.
- If the GP is willing to prescribe an unfamiliar treatment, or one being used outside its licence:
  Dosage and administration should be specified by a consultant.
  For unlicensed uses, a full justification should be provided.
  A treatment protocol should be provided.

Over-the-counter medicines (OTCs)

About 20% of the £4500m spent each year in the UK on medicines is on OTCs.[32] Prescription-only medicines (PoM) can only be got with a prescription. Pharmacy (P) medicines can only be got from a pharmacy with a pharmacist in attendance. Other medicines are on general sale.

In the interests of economy and reducing NHS workload, the government is encouraging more people to self-medicate for minor illness. Community pharmacists are trained to offer advice on drugs, self-medication, and when a doctor should be consulted.

On the other hand, concerns are expressed that serious illness may go undiagnosed, and some OTC preparations may interact with other OTCs or prescribed treatments.

The GP is bound by terms and conditions of service to provide a prescription for any medication which he or she recommends for a patient he or she is treating. For the 20% or so of prescriptions which are not exempt from charge, the cost of the medicine may be less than the prescription charge (currently £4.75).

For OTC or P medicines, the patient can be given a prescription, and informed that the cost direct from the pharmacist may be less than a prescription charge. For PoM medicines, a prescription has to be issued. It is now allowable to issue private prescriptions to list patients if the cost of the medication is less than the prescription charge.

References

1. George C. Introducing PILS. *MIMS* 1988; **15**: 75–80
2. Gilley J. Towards rational prescribing. *Br Med J* 1994; **308**: 731–2
3. Fry J. Factfile on prescribing. *Update* 1993; **47**: 697
4. *Pharmaceutical Briefing 6*. London: Association of British Pharmaceutical Industries. 1989
5. *Working for Patients*. London: Association of British Pharmaceutical Industries. 1989
6. Roberts SJ and Harris CM. Age, sex and temporary resident originated prescribing units (ASTRO-PUs). *Br Med J* 1993; **307**: 485–8
7. Knox JDE. The five elements that make for noncompliance. *Modern Med* 1989; 391–4
8. George CF. How to get your patients to take their medicine. *Update* 1994; **48**: 519–23
9. Beardon PHG, McGilchrist MM, McKendrick AD *et al*. Primary non-compliance with prescribed medication in primary care. *Br Med J* 1993; **307**: 846–8
10. George CF. What do patients need to know about prescribed drugs? *Prescribers' J* 1994; **34**: 7–11
11. User leaflets. *Br Med J* 1990; **300**: 420
12. Aronson JK and Hardman M. Patient compliance. *Br Med J* 1992; **305**: 1009–11
13. How drugs get to market. *Drug Ther Bull* 1990; **28**: 24
14. Harry J. Discovery and development of a new drug. *Prescribers' J* 1991; **31**: 221–26
15. Smith R. Drug innovation in Britain. *Br Med J* 1988; **297**: 1152
16. New terms for the pharmaceutical price regulation scheme. *Drug Ther Bull* 1993; **31**: 20
17. Smith R. Doctors and the drug industry: too close for comfort. *Br Med J* 1986; **293**: 905–6
18. *Guidelines on Postmarketing Surveillance*. Joint Committee of ABPI, BMA, CSM and RCGP. London 1990 – Authors are a committee formed from the quoted organizations
19. *Prescribing and Cost Analysis Level 1*. 1993; London: Prescription Pricing Authority
20. Loshak D. Are generics a bargain? *Med Monitor* 1989; **2**, 6–7
21. Generic prescribing. *MeReC Bull* 1991; **2**: 22–24
22. Parallel imported medicines. *MeRec Bull* 1991; **2**: 39–40
23. Van Zwanenberg T. How to cut your drugs bill. *MIMS* 1989; **16**: 27–31
24. Economic prescribing. *Drug Ther Bull* 1991; **29**: 5–7
25. Hepburn A. The interpretation and use of PACT. *Prescribers' J* 1991; **31**: 49–56

26. Stott P. Formularies – friend or foe? *Horizons* 1992; **6**: 542–4
27. Slaiman S. Formularies are an unwanted necessity. *MIMS* 1990; **17**: 21
28. Schutte PK. Some legal considerations in prescribing. *Prescribers' J* 1991; **31**: 27–33
29. British Medical Association. *Second GMSC Guidance on Product Liability*. London: BMA. 1988
30. Prescribing unlicensed drugs or using drugs for unlicensed indications. *Drug Ther Bull* 1992; **30**: 97–99
31. Department of Health. *Responsibilities for Prescribing between Hospitals and GPs*. EL(91)127. London: HMSO. 1991
32. Medicines without an NHS prescription. *Drug Ther Bull* 1994; **32**: 4–5

16

Membership examination for the Royal College of General Practitioners (MRCGP)

Aims

The trainee should:

- Know the format of the MRCGP examination.
- Be able to decide whether or not to take the examination.
- Be able to assess written material critically.

Why take the MRCGP?

The Royal College of General Practitioners (RCGP) was founded in 1952. In 1965 the first membership exam was held. Five people took it and they all passed. By 1968 all new college members had to have passed the exam, and this situation has pertained since.

The exam may be taken in May or October. Now about 2000 candidates sit the exam each year. These are mainly trainees or those who have recently completed vocational training, so that about 80% of trainees sit the exam. Currently around half of all GPs are college members, and this figure will surely rise with time.

The overall pass rate of the exam is now around 75%. Different categories of candidate have different pass rates. If you are a British-born woman graduate of a British medical school who has just finished vocational training and who is sitting the exam for the first time, then your chance of passing is well over 90%. On the other hand, experienced male overseas graduates taking the exam for the fourth time can save themselves the entrance fee (£295 in 1994) by not bothering.

Trainees sit the exam for three main reasons:[1]

1. To help get a job – 71%.
2. To provide discipline in vocational training – 67%.

3. To ensure a basic level of competence before working unsupervised – 66%.

In addition, holding the MRCGP is now required in many regions in order to be approved as a GP trainer. Anyone wishing to become an examiner for the college has to resit the exam.

Strenuous efforts are made to ensure that the exam is a valid reflection of competence as a GP, but this has yet to be proven. It is very difficult to measure competence objectively, and there are probably as many versions of what constitutes competence as there are GPs. On the other hand, the MRCGP is at present the only British postgraduate exam which even attempts to examine overall competence as a GP.

For a population wanting a high-quality service, and a government anxious to ensure it is getting good value for the large sums it is investing in vocational training, the discrepancy between the pass rate of the MRCGP and the pass rate for vocational training programmes (over 99%) is of concern. From 1996, all trainees will be subject to a compulsory summative assessment at the end of their training, and it is widely estimated that a failure rate of about 5% is being expected from this.

The college is keen that their exam should be used as the end-point assessment, and they clearly have more expertise in setting an exam of this kind than anybody else. The counterargument runs that not everyone supports what the college stands for, and would not want to be associated with it. In addition, the standards of the exam would have to be altered.

How do you enter for the exam?

Certain criteria have to be satisfied before you can take the exam.

1. You must be a fully registered medical practitioner and have 3 years' postregistration experience (full-time or the equivalent part-time). Many trainees will not have finished their full 3 years at the time they want to take the exam, and in this case their application has to be endorsed by the postgraduate dean, regional adviser or course organizer.
2. You must pay the entrance fee. This is not redeemable if you fail.
3. You must hold a certificate of competence in cardiopulmonary resuscitation. There is usually a fee to be met from whoever makes the assessment and provides the certificate. Ambulance departments are usually quite happy to arrange this.

4. You must hold a certificate of competence in child health surveillance. This can be done through your trainer (if on the child health surveillance list) or a paediatrician.

Details of these last two criteria are sent together with the application forms to sit the exam.

Candidates are also asked to complete a practice experience questionnaire to be sent to the college 4 or 5 weeks before the oral part of the exam. This is not marked, but provides a basis for questions at one of the orals. The pro forma for this is sent with the application forms.

What form does the exam take?

The exam is taken on two separate days, several weeks apart. There are five parts, three written and two oral. Each part carries 20% of the final marks. All the written parts are done on the first day, and this can make for a very strenuous experience if you have spent the last 4 years writing only brief notes with lots of abbreviations and no punctuation. The written papers are marked first, and the top 85% of candidates then go on to sit the orals.

The written papers are peer-referenced so that always 85% of candidates proceed to the orals. You don't get an oral unless you pass the written. The orals used to be criterion-referenced to try and achieve the same standard for each block of candidates. This has now stopped, and the entire exam is peer-referenced. The pass rate is thus decided in advance.

The results of the different papers all have a different mean and standard deviation. The crude results are revised so as to create a standard distribution where the rank order of the candidates is the same as for the original marks. To achieve this, very well or very badly answered questions may be not counted in the final total. A score of under 37.5% will fail; 47.5% is average. A score of 57.5% will place you in the top seventh of candidates.

Each candidate is notified of his or her scores. Those who fail also receive a detailed critique of their performance.

The written exam can be taken in any one of 12 venues, one of which is in Germany. The orals are held in London and Edinburgh.

The multiple choice questionnaire (MCQ)

This is the most enduring part of the exam, and of all the parts of the exam correlates most closely with the overall result. It tests only knowledge, but is exceptionally good at it. A reliability coefficient (that is, the ratio of scores if the same candidate is tested on two separate occasions) of 0.84 is currently being achieved.[2] A store of questions is held by the college, and each exam is a combination of new and old questions, about 75% of questions having been used before. The trial questions are distributed randomly, and the results are not counted in the candidate's mark. Questions are devised with reference to authoritative sources, particularly *Update* and *Medicine International*. All answers are validated from at least two separate sources. The MCQ panel recommends as preparation for the MCQ that candidates read the *British Medical Journal*, the *British Journal of General Practice*, the *British National Formulary* and the *Drug and Therapeutics Bulletin*. Additionally, the candidate with plenty of free time could look at *The Practitioner, Update, Medicine International* and MRCGP publications.[2]

Every effort is made so that questions are not ambiguous, and there are some standard phrases used:

- *Characteristic* implies a feature of diagnostic significance whose absence would cast doubt on the diagnosis.
- *Typical* implies a feature whose presence would be expected but is perhaps not as diagnostically absolute as characteristic.
- *Recognized* implies a fact which has been reliably reported and which a candidate would be expected to know, without the fact being necessarily characteristic or typical.
- *Has been shown* implies information which has been repeated so often as to gain the accolade of accepted truth or could be demonstrated by reference to an authoritative paper on the subject.

The questions are answered on a marking grid for easy computer analysis. There are 2 hours allowed for the paper.

Wrong answers were negatively marked until 1992, but not now. Apparently negative marking encourages guesses, and some people guess better than others. Negative marking selects against candidates from overseas, and particularly women. Most postgraduate medical exams contain an MCQ, and many have now stopped negative marking for the same reasons.

There are a number of traditional MCQ questions. For each of these there is a stem with a number of items deriving from it, usually 4–6. The total number of items is always 360.

Questions are all mixed up, but follow this approximate distribution:

Medicine	60
Therapeutics	36
Surgical diagnosis	18
Physical medicine/trauma	18
Infectious diseases	12
Care of the elderly	12
Paediatrics	30
Obstetrics/gynaecology	36
Psychiatry	36
Dermatology	24
Ophthalmology	18
Ear, nose and throat	12
Ethical/legal	12
Epidemiology/research method	12
Practice organization	24

In addition, there are some extended matching questions (EMQs). These are intended to assess diagnostic pattern recognition. A list of diagnostic options is matched to a list of case scenarios, with only one option each to be selected.

The modified essay question (MEQ) paper

The MEQ is designed to test decision-making skills. It will also test attitudes to a degree, and possibly a little knowledge, but this is not its aim.

Two hours are allowed. You are given usually 10 but up to 12 scenarios which are usually adaptations of true case histories, and asked to answer a question about them. Two or more scenarios can be linked as an ongoing case, and in fact the paper used to consist entirely of an evolving case in 10 parts. These proved too difficult to devise.

In particular, the examiners are looking for:[3]

- Straightforward clinical decision-making skills.
- Management of chronic conditions.
- Management of difficult patients.
- Dealing with psychological problems.
- Knowledge of family dynamics.
- Evidence of consultation skills.
- Ability to work with colleagues.
- Awareness of practice management issues.
- Knowledge of ethical considerations.

- Dealing with controversial topics.
- The doctor's own feelings.

When constructing an answer, think in terms of:

- Physical/psychological/social.
- Doctor/patient/community.
- Explore/explain/act.
- Doctor/partners/staff.
- Advantages/disadvantages. Questions starting 'Discuss ...'.
- Positive/negative.

The examiners are looking for breadth of knowledge. You should aim to cover as many different aspects as you can. Short notes are best. Headings, underlining and highlighting are perfectly all right. The examiner has about 90 seconds to mark each question – each is marked by a separate examiner – so legible handwriting is essential.

You only have about 10 minutes per question, so don't hang about. You need to write about one side of A4 per answer and there should be enough substance in the question to do this.

This paper is construct-marked. The group of examiners responsible for the paper meet and identify separate areas of knowledge or constructs to which the answer should refer. Four to 10 constructs will be identified per question. Five marks are allocated to each. An average pre-adjusted mark would be 20–25 out of 45.

Examples of constructs would be:[4]

- Clinical competence.
- Consultation skills.
- Awareness of patient's hidden agenda.
- Recognition of the patient's point of view.
- Ability to predict future developments.
- Cost-effectiveness.
- Follow-up arrangements.
- Insight into family or social influences on outcome.
- Preventive interventions.
- Financial and business acumen.
- Awareness of ethical considerations.
- Involvement of other team members.
- Awareness of doctor's own feelings and motivations.
- Clinical safety.
- *Caritas* – sense of genuine caring or empathy.
- Logical and systematic approach.

The critical reading question (CRQ)

This is the latest part of the exam to be introduced, and makes most candidates go weak at the knees. Since its introduction in 1990 it has already undergone significant changes in structure, and so what follows applies to the situation at May 1994.

This paper tests knowledge to some degree, but is mainly looking at problem-solving skills and attitudes. It aims to assess the ability to evaluate critically published material and other data to inform general practice decision-making. There are two sections to the paper and $2\frac{1}{2}$ hours are allowed.

Reading and current practice

There are five questions on topics of current interest. It is often possible to spot likely topics and read accordingly. The major important issues like hypertension, depression and diabetes are always possible. Also remember that the paper is set in December/January for the following May and October, so consider the 'hot topics' around at that time. Review articles from the *British Journal of General Practice* are particularly significant. More ideas can be gleaned from the RCGP *Handbooks*: all the questions one year were based on this source.

It is hard to know how much needs to be included about specific references, and it is this issue which scares many trainees. Quoting from a recent college publication:[5]

> The majority of the marks available will be awarded for demonstrating an *understanding* [my italics] of the current views and research. Candidates should try and indicate the source of the evidence and views which they present.

If what you put down is sound practice, then you will pass, and any references should be seen as the icing on the cake. If you can produce one or two references per topic, that is more than adequate.

Critical appraisal

You are given five pieces of written material to evaluate and interpret critically. The material may be published papers or extracts from papers such as summaries or methods and results sections on their own. It may also include data relevant to general practice such as a protocol, a report, an audit or a series of clinical results. The type of material will be varied.

The papers used so far have all been from the *British Medical Journal* or the *British Journal of General Practice*, and published within the last 5 years. For copyright reasons this is unlikely to change. There is always something in the paper to criticize, but not too much, bearing in mind that they will all have been refereed before publication.

How can you assess papers?

Writing a summary

If you are asked to produce a summary for a paper, it should contain the following four elements:[6]

1. *Objectives.* What are the authors really trying to measure? The more succinct the objectives, the better.
2. *Design.* There are basically six types of design:
   a. Case report – an interesting or unusual case.
   b. Case series – a description of several cases.
   c. Cross-sectional study – a snapshot view of a disease, factor or characteristic at a point in time.
   d. Cohort study – monitoring a group for events over time.
   e. Case control study – comparing people with a disease with another group without the disease.
   f. Controlled trial – comparing the results from two matched groups, one with and one without a specified intervention.
3. *Important results.*
4. *Authors' conclusions.*

Assessing objectives and design

A series of six questions can be applied which will bring out the important features:[6]

1. Is the study design appropriate to the objectives? This is largely a matter of common sense. For instance, a study comparing treatments has to be a controlled trial.
2. Is the study sample representative?
   a. The sample group should be typical and representative of the group for whom the research is likely to influence care.
   b. The sampling method must be random so that no group is over- or underrepresented.

c. The sample size must be sufficient to make the conclusions valid. A very slight effect can only be confirmed from large numbers of subjects, otherwise the confidence limits are too wide.

d. The study sample should not exclude, by entry criteria or by drop-outs, groups of subjects who might have their care influenced by the study. The entry criteria should not exclude the subjects with whom you are most likely to be dealing. One way of resolving the drop-out problem is to use intention to treat. In this method, all the subjects recruited are followed up, not just those who fully complete the intervention under investigation.

e. Are the drop-outs or non-responders likely to give you the same answers as the study group? What efforts have been made to ensure that data are obtained from as many subjects in the original study group as possible?

3. Is the control group acceptable? The control group should be matched for all the factors which are known to influence the study topic. For instance, a study on heart attack should match for age, sex and cigarette smoking in the control group. The thoroughness of the controlling process depends on previous knowledge of other research in the field.

4. Is the quality of measurement and outcome adequate? A number of areas can be looked at:

a. *Validity.* Do the measurements measure what they are supposed to measure? It is common to use surrogate measures for disease rather than the disease itself. A common example is the use of changes in serum lipid profile as a proxy for heart attacks.

b. *Reliability.* Are the same results likely at a different time with a different observer.

c. *Blindness.* Could the wishes of the researchers to get an 'interesting result' have influenced the study? Could the wishes of the subjects to cooperate have influenced their reports of symptoms?

d. *Quality.* Is there sufficient attention to quality issues? Results based on observer assessment are likely to be less reliable than those based on laboratory results or using assessment protocols.

5. Is the study complete? If there are too many drop-outs, then this increases the chance that the drop-out group will give different results from the reported group. Attention might be given to:

a. Compliance. This can be overcome by the intention to treat method.

b. Drop-outs and deaths.
c. Missing data.
6. Is the control group free of distortion? It is best if as many confounding factors as possible are controlled for. In addition, the analysis technique should allow for any factors which are only recognized when the research data have been collected.

Distorting factors include:

a. Controls may have tried other treatment for the same condition – a confounding factor termed extraneous treatment.
b. The controls may have been affected by the study group – so-called contamination.
c. The passage of time may have altered the controls.

Making a final judgement

All research can be criticized. Research is easier to criticize than to perform. Using the above criteria, a balance still has to be weighed: shall I believe this evidence or not.

Bias
Have the results been biased in some way? This may not invalidate the work if the bias has been recognized and allowed for.

Confounding factors
Are there serious distorting influences?

Chance
What is the likelihood that the results arose by chance? Attention to adequate statistical method should prevent this. The use of the 5% confidence limit (that is, a P value of 0.05) is arbitrary, but has become the established norm. This means, however, that using these limits there is still a 1 in 20 chance that any changes have happened by chance.

The oral examinations

There are two 30-minute orals with a 5-minute gap. There are two examiners for each part.

Eighty-five per cent of candidates get an oral, and you only get an oral if you pass the written papers. You have to pass both written and orals to pass the exam. The orals are now peer-referenced.

Orals test some knowledge, but mainly skills and attitudes. It is the only part of the exam to test interview skills.

First oral

This is based on the practice experience questionnaire which is filled in beforehand and sent to the examiners. It is important to keep a copy for reference. The information required includes personal data, practice structure, organization and facilities, workload, the candidate's own ideas and learning experiences, and a clinical diary of 25 surgery consultations, 15 home visits and 10 emergency calls. Some of the details needed may not be readily to hand, and the time to fill it in may be short.

At each oral, six topics will be discussed for 5 minutes each. Seven areas of competence will be examined in each oral:[1]

Problem definition
Application of knowledge. Recognizing the whole problem. Applying probabilities. Consider options. Critical thinking.

Management
Whole-patient care. Life-threatening problems. Chronic diseases. Psychological problems. Use of resources. Prescribing.

Prevention
Preventive medicine. Health education.

Practice organization
Accessibility. Team work. Time management. Priorities.

Communication
Doctor–patient communication. Patients' health beliefs.

Professional values
Respect for life. Responsibility and reliability. Respect for people. Empathy and sensitivity. Integrity and ethics. Enjoyment and enthusiasm.

Personal and professional growth
Self-awareness. Personal/professional balances. Self-assessment. Reading and literature. Continued education.

In the answers, the examiners will be looking for evidence of:

- Coherence.
- Rationality.
- Consistency.
- Justification of behaviour, opinions and attitudes.
- Attitudes and behaviour consistent with practice.

The second oral

This is the so-called problem-solving viva. A series of clinical or other scenarios will be presented for comment. The same areas of competence are being examined as in the first oral, but you will have no warning as to what topics might come up. Much of it will consist of issues you have not considered before, and so a certain amount of 'thinking on your feet' is required. It is all right to say if you don't know an answer, and better this than to dig a hole for yourself, from which it may be difficult to climb.

Preparing for the exam

It will be necessary to make the decision to enter for the exam between 6 and 12 months beforehand. This will give enough time for preparation. The factual knowledge required is significant. In addition, the exam seeks to assess for an attitude of mind consistent with current good general practice.

Find out about the exam

Many postgraduate centres run a preparation course for candidates. Try and choose one which involves college examiners as a resource. Gaining insight into their thinking can be most useful. Considerable efforts are made to ensure the consistency of the examiners. The course should also give you a chance to do some mock papers and orals in a situation where they can be peer-reviewed, so you will know whether or not you are with the pace.

Do some practice papers

You will be sent some past papers with the exam application forms. It is worth doing a few of these under exam conditions beforehand. They can then be reviewed with your trainer or your peers.

Join an exam preparation group

Candidates often find it useful to meet with other candidates on a regular basis. Meetings can be to review mock papers, to share insight and useful information/references on 'hot topics', and to offer mutual support.

Undertake a reading programme

It is important to know what to read. It is even more important to know what not to read. There are an estimated 30 000 biomedical journals in the world, a number which has been growing by 7% a year since the 17th century. However, it is also estimated that only 15% of medical interventions are supported by solid scientific evidence.[7] The ability to read wisely and with discrimination is not only important to pass the exam, it is also a necessary technique to apply to all your future professional reading.

When deciding if a piece is worth reading, the following guidelines have been suggested:[8]

1. Is the paper relevant to my work?
2. Will the paper tell me something I don't already know?
3. Can the information in the paper be applied to the group of patients I am likely to see?
4. Can the evidence be believed? Is the research of an acceptably high standard?

For the purposes of the exam, it is reasonable to read only a small number of journals. A suitable list would be:

British Medical Journal.
British Journal of General Practice.
Update.
British National Formulary.
Drug and Therapeutics Bulletin.

Attend the day-release course regularly

Most trainees and GPs will have a nearby vocational training scheme which runs a half-day course each week. The topics for these will be chosen by the trainees and the course organizers as relevant to training. Meeting doctors of like mind is a good way of making sure that your attitudes and knowledge are not too far away from normal.

You may very well hold beliefs which are not orthodox, and it can be argued that only by challenging orthodoxy can progress be made. In professional life, as in the MRCGP exam, unorthodox beliefs should be supported by evidence. The regular re-examination of beliefs is an important part of the ongoing education of all GPs.

References

1. MRCGP guide. *GP Newspaper* April 29 1994; 83–6
2. Turner J. Passing the MRCGP: the MCQ. *The Practitioner* 1993; **237**: 836–39
3. Wilson A. Passing the MRCGP: the MEQ. *The Practitioner* 1993; **237**: 913–16
4. Neighbour R. *Construct Marking – the MEQ Examiner's Vade Mecum.* London: Royal College of General Practitioners. 1992
5. Examination for membership. RCGP Connection March 1994. Journal Supplement to *Br J. Gen Pract* **44**: 1–11
6. Fowkes FGR & Fulton PM. Critical appraisal of published research. Introductory guidelines. *Br Med J* 1991; **302**: 1136–40
7. Smith R. Where is the wisdom ...? *Br Med J* 1991; **303**: 798–9
8. Macauley D. READER: an acronym to aid critical reading by general practitioners. *Br J Gen Pract* 1994; **44**: 83–5

Index